From Bench to Bedside, to Track & Field

The Context of Enhancement and its Ethical Relevance

Perspectives in Medical Humanities

Perspectives in Medical Humanities publishes peer reviewed scholarship produced or reviewed under the auspices of the University of California Medical Humanities Consortium, a multi-campus collaborative of faculty, students, and trainees in the humanities, medicine, and health sciences. Our series invites scholars from the humanities and health care professions to share narratives and analysis on health, healing, and the contexts of our beliefs and practices that impact biomedical inquiry.

General Editor

Brian Dolan, PhD, Professor of Social Medicine and Medical Humanities, University of California, San Francisco (UCSF)

Recent Titles

Clowns and Jokers Can Heal Us: Comedy and Medicine
By Albert Howard Carter III (Fall 2011)

The Remarkables: Endocrine Abnormalities in Art
By Carol Clark and Orlo Clark (Winter 2011)

Health Citizenship: Essays in Social Medicine and Biomedical Politics
By Dorothy Porter (Winter 2011)

What to Read on Love, Not Sex: Freud, Fiction, and the Articulation of Truth in Modern Psychological Science
By Edison Miyawaki, MD, Foreword by Harold Bloom (Fall 2012)

Patient Poets: Illness from Inside Out
Marilyn Chandler McEntyre (Fall 2012) (Pedagogy in Medical Humanities series)

Bioethics and Medical Issues in Literature
Mahala Yates Stripling (Fall 2013) (Pedagogy in Medical Humanities series)

www.UCMedicalHumanitiesPress.com

This series is made possible by the generous support of the Dean of the School of Medicine at UCSF, the Center for Humanities and Health Sciences at UCSF, and a Multicampus Research Program Grant from the University of California Office of the President.

From Bench to Bedside, to Track & Field

The Context of Enhancement and its Ethical Relevance

Silvia Camporesi

First published in 2014

by University of California Medical Humanities Press

in partnership with eScholarship | University of California

© 2014 by Silvia Camporesi

University of California

Medical Humanities Consortium

3333 California Street, Suite 485

San Francisco, CA 94143-0850

Cover image used with permission:

Vladimir Veličković, Belgrado, 1935. Depart (Figura di Atleta Nudo in Partenza) 1973

Acrilico tecnica mista su tela, 146x198 cm.

Inv n. 1783

Palazzo Romagnoli Forlì, Collezioni del Novecento

Book design by Virtuoso Press.

Library of Congress Control Number: 2014934965

ISBN: 978-0-9889865-4-1

Printed in USA

Table of Contents

Acknowledgments

This book builds to a large extent on my PhD dissertation in Philosophy of Medicine for King's College London, in particular chapters 1-3, which have been revised and elaborated since the viva in October 2013. Chapter 4 includes new material, while part of the content that was in my PhD thesis has been left out to improve readability of this work.

I am deeply grateful to my supervisor, Dr Matteo Mameli, Reader in Philosophy at King's College London, for supporting and mentoring me, and allowing me a wide degree of freedom in pursuing my research interests during my PhD. I would also like to acknowledge the Wellcome Trust for funding my PhD, and Professor Richard Ashcroft from Queen Mary University and Søren Holm from the University of Manchester for being my PhD examiners and helping me substantially improve this work through their valuable insights and feedback.

From 2010 to 2013 I had the privilege of working in the intellectually stimulating atmosphere of the Wellcome Trust-funded Centre for the Humanities & Health at King's College London. I am grateful to all my colleagues at the Centre for the engaging discussions on medical humanities and philosophy of medicine (among other topics!) over the past three years. In particular, thanks to Elisabetta Babini, Natalie Banner, Monika Class, Bonnie Evans, Keren Hammerschlag, Elselijn Kingma, MM McCabe, David Papineau, Anne Marie Rafferty, Maria Vaccarella, and Stefan Wagner. Thanks goes to Professor Brian Hurwitz, Director of the Centre, for being a great counselor on many fronts and several occasions, and for his great support in helping me launch my career. I now have the pleasure of working in the recently established Department of Social Science, Health & Medicine at King's College London, and I thank Professor Nikolas Rose, Head of Department, and all my new colleagues at SSHM for welcoming me and fostering such a vibrant environment.

This work is also to a good extent the result of work I conducted as a visiting PhD student at the Department of Anthropology, History and Social Medicine (DAHSM) at University of California, San Francisco in 2011/12. I am most grateful first and foremost to Professor Dorothy Porter, and then to all the members of the department, for welcoming me and giving me so many research and work opportunities during my year as a visiting scholar there. A special thanks goes to Brian Dolan, Director of UC Medical Humanities Consortium, for his encouragement and for his inestimable work as Editor of the Perspectives in Medical Humanities Series.

Since 2011 Professor Mike McNamee from the University of Swansea has been an invaluable collaborator and mentor. This work incorporates one of our co-authored papers in section 3.2 and references two other co-authored papers. Many thanks go also to my co-author Paolo Maugeri for our long discussions on the Caster Semenya case, and for giving me permission to include a portion of our co-authored article in this work (section 4.4).

I am very grateful to my husband James Knuckles for also granting me permission to include a portion of our paper in this work (sections 4.1 and 4.2), and in addition for his invaluable patience, support and encouragement over the writing of my PhD thesis. I gratefully acknowledge permission from Cambridge University Press, Taylor & Francis, Springer and Routledge to reproduce portions of articles in revised form in this book (sections 2.4, 3.2, 3.4., 4.1 and 4.2; publisher and co-authors also acknowledged as footnotes in the text). I also acknowledge Dr Cristina Ambrosini, Director of Art Museums in Forlì, for granting me permission to use the work "Figura di atleta nudo in partenza" by Vladimir Veličković for the cover image of this book.

I would also like to acknowledge Mauro Giacca, Director of the International Centre for Genetic Engineering and Biotechnology and former mentor, and Matt Springer at UCSF, for their expert opinions on gene enhancement; and Lisa Bortolotti, Professor of Philosophy at the University of Birmingham, for her constant support and encouragement throughout the years, and for being my role model of a successful academic, woman and mother.

Last but not least, my deepest thanks go to my family, whose unwavering support over the years has given me the greatest gift: the freedom to pursue my interests.

Foreword

Professor Søren Holm
Manchester University & University of Oslo & Aalborg University

The "enhancement debate," i.e. the academic discussion of whether physical or cognitive enhancement of human beings is ethically acceptable or not, is often conducted with no real engagement between the protagonists on each side. Each side has its own set of stock arguments, counterarguments and cases (often hypothetical or highly idealised), that in most cases fail to engage in any meaningful way with the ethical concerns that motivate the other side in the debate. As a reader of the enhancement debate it is easy to become bored because the debate does not really seem to be moving, each side just reiterating its original position with ever more elaborate arguments.

This book is, however, a fine example of how the debate can move forward if the protagonists were really interested in engaging with the question of whether or not a particular set of enhancements should be promoted, allowed or prohibited in a particular context. The approach taken by Silvia Camporesi is casuistic in the sense that it takes its point of departure not in some idealised philosophical question, e.g. is there a sustainable distinction between treatment and enhancement, but in concrete, specific cases. The analysis is philosophically rigorous, but each of the cases she considers is considered with due attention to all its complexity and to how it is similar, but yet different from other enhancement cases. This is definitely not armchair philosophising, but applied ethics as it should be done.

Reading the book leads to the interesting realisation that a casuistic approach does not preclude new and generalisable conclusions. In analysing a range of cases in detail Dr. Camporesi shows that we can reach firm conclusions about many aspects of the individual cases, although these conclusions often have to be more carefully caveated than is usually done in the enhancement debate. But we can also reach some new, interesting and quite general conclusions, for instance about the need to allow research into enhancement technologies, even in cases where we are still unsure whether a particular type of putative enhancement is ethically acceptable or not.

A further major contribution that is made in this book is to press the point that it is a mistake to conflate ethical and policy issues. Our ethical analysis may in the best of circumstances provide us with an answer to whether a particular enhancement that is desired by a particular person, in a particular context is ethically acceptable or not, but it rarely provides an answer to the question of what policy a particular society should adopt in relation to enhancements of this particular type. The equality implications of promoting, allowing or prohibiting a particular type of enhancement may for instance vary immensely between different societies and this will have implication for what policy a society ought to pursue. So, as soon as we move from the level of ethics to the level of policy we need not only to engage with ethical theory but also with political philosophy. Camporesi expresses this much better than I can:

> Moral disagreement in society will persist, no matter what philosophers may say. This, however, is not an indication of the fact that all views in the field of philosophical ethics are equivalent or incommensurable. Rather, it high-lights how, in practice, we face a political problem. The pressing questions posed by genethics do not allow us simply to acknowledge that moral positions differ and then nonconfrontationally to concern ourselves with ironing out internal inconsistencies. Instead, they demand a shift in focus from classical philosophical ethics to the realm of political philosophy. (p. 130)

If every participant in the "enhancement debate" took this to heart, and attended to the messy reality of introducing any kind of enhancement in the real world to the same degree as the author of this book, then there would perhaps be hope that we could move on from the current stylised, stale and largely hypothetical non-debate that characterises the literature.

Introduction

This book addresses the issue of human enhancement technologies and their ethical permissibility through a contextual, bottom up approach based on case studies. The first chapter familiarizes the reader with the various definitions that have been put forward for "enhancement," and the arguments for and against. I then argue in favour of a neutral definition of enhancement, where decisions regarding the ethical permissibility of a technology are reached through a contextual analysis aimed at spelling out the values intrinsic in the particular practice under scrutiny. In this first chapter I also discuss the value of distinguishing therapy versus enhancement, and distinguishing absolute versus positional goods.

In the second chapter I discuss the application of genetic technologies from the "bench" (of research on molecular biology) to the "bedside" of clinical trials and experimentation on pharmaceuticals on human beings.

The first part of the chapter is dedicated to the discussion of the objections to genetic technologies aimed at enhancing human capacities and grounded in the resurgence of "eugenics." To answer the question of whether the ethical objections against classical eugenics are still valid against contemporary practices of reproductive genetic choices, I provide a comparative historical overview of eugenics in the UK, the US and Scandinavia. I divide the analysis into three periods: (a) "classical eugenics" (1883-1945), (b) "modern eugenics," from the end of WW II to the first 'test tube baby' (1946-1978), and (c) "contemporary eugenics," from the birth of Louise Brown until now (1978-2014). I highlight similarities and differences between the three periods and address whether the ethical objections to classical and modern eugenics are still valid today, and whether the contemporary use of genetic technologies in the reproductive context to choose children's traits can still be called "eugenics."

The second part of the chapter is dedicated to the analysis of how pre-implantation genetic diagnosis and other genetic screening techniques at the level of the human embryo raise a conflict of interest between parental re-productive freedom and children's right to an open future and capacity for self-determination. As a case study, in section 2.4 I analyse the case of parents choosing to have deaf children through pre-implantation genetic diagnosis. The expressivist argument that deafness (or other traits traditionally considered disabilities) is "only a difference" is the focus of my analysis in section 2.5.

Genetic technologies impact all stages of life, and in Chapter 3 I analyse how genetic technologies, and in particular gene transfer, are translated direct-ly from the molecular genetics/biology laboratory to "track & field," where they are applied with the goal of enhancing athletic performance, without going through the clinical research step of experimentation of the pharma-ceuticals in human subjects.

In the first part of chapter 3 I discuss gene transfer technologies applied to enhance athletic performance. In section 3.1 I analyse the scientific and reg-ulatory context of gene enhancement, and the basis on which these technolo-gies are classified as doping. In section 3.2 I focus my analysis on a real case study of a gene transfer clinical trial aimed at raising tolerance to pain, and discuss its ethical permissibility in therapeutic and professional sport contexts.

In the second part of the chapter (sections 3.3 and 3.4) I discuss the ethi-cal and social implications of the recent boom in direct-to-consumer genetic tests to scout out children's athletic potential. In the last section of the chapter I discuss performance enhancement and anti-doping governance, and analyse the arguments in favour of introducing doping in sport under a controlled and regulated medical context.

In Chapter 4 I discuss how professional sport has always been a laboratory for biomedical and biotechnological innovations regarding the treatment of injury, recovery and training regimes aimed at maximising athletic performance. It is a matter of fact that elite athletes are willing to accept high degrees of risk in exchange for the expected performance enhancing benefits derived from the consumption of prohibited substances, from extreme training regimes or diets, or the experimentation upon themselves of innovative surgeries. In the first part of the chapter (sections 4.1 and 4.2) I propose an alternative way to alter the practice of high-performance athletes discounting future health for current performance, without engaging in doping under a medical context, by shifting the burden of proof from the regulator to the sponsors, as well as providing the right incentives in the form of penalties to the sponsors whose athletes test positive. In order to do so, I borrow arguments from similar discussions in the sustainability field, where it has long been proposed to shift the burden of proof of damaging the environment from regulators to the private sector. In the second part of the chapter (section 4.3) I tackle the broader question of an ethical justification for research on enhancement, which has been surprisingly neglected in the bioethical debate on enhancement. I argue that even though particular technologies aimed at enhancing human capacities are not ethically permissible in a certain context, it does not follow that research on enhancement *per se* is also not ethically permissible.

Moral disagreement in society about bioethical issues will persist, no matter what philosophical arguments are put forward. The pressing questions posed by enhancement technologies do not allow us simply to acknowledge that moral positions differ and then nonconfrontationally concern ourselves with ironing out internal inconsistencies in the different positions. Rather, they demand a shift in focus from classical philosophical ethics to the realm of political philosophy. This is what I try to do in the last section of chapter 4, where I lay the groundwork for the discussion of how to shift the debate on enhancement technology from the ethical level to a policy level, and to analyse the role for the philosopher in the enhancement debate.

All throughout this work I adopt a casuistic approach to ethics, meaning I deploy different tools from deontologist, consequentialist, principled and virtue-ethics approaches, trying to bring the debate on enhancement out of the stalemate caused by the polarization of proponents and opponents. In each case I discuss the ethical permissibility of a technology in a way that could be used to inform policymaking, and to bring forward the bioethical debate in a productive way. I am aware that the work contained in this book is preliminary and incomplete, but I hope that it will point towards interesting and original directions for research, for example at the intersection of sport, medicine and ethics, where traditional ethical issues in clinical research are exacerbated in the context of elite sports; and in the field of reprogenetics, where the use of genetic technologies to choose children's traits traditionally considered a disability force us to rethink the debate surrounding enhancement and the resurgence of eugenics.

Chapter One

Framing the ethical debate on enhancement technologies

1.1 What we talk about when we talk about "enhancement"

> Because human enhancement apparently involves altering human nature, it is meant to be the sort of thing that sends shivers down the spine. For 'transhumanists,' these are frissons of excitement at the thought of a wonderful new world of genetically and pharmaceutically augmented, ultra-intelligent, long-lived super-persons. For conservatives such as Leon Kass, our shivers are the wise verdict of an instinctive moral repugnance. (Lewens 2009, 354)

It is a matter of fact that the mere mention of the possibility of "human enhancement" is able to spark a vehement discussion between staunch supporters and vocal opponents.. Lewens is quite right in putting the finger on the instinctive opposite reactions triggered by the newest possibilities opened by biomedical enhancements. But what exactly is so unique about human enhancement that is able to elicit such visceral reactions? It seems to be the perception that human enhancement technologies are tinkering with human nature, and that humans engaging with biomedical enhancements are playing at projects of self-creation and self-evolution that are hubristic and may lead to dangerous slippery slopes. Before addressing the arguments on both sides, a disclaimer is necessary: both reactions described above are extreme examples triggered by misrepresentation of the real scientifically feasible prospects of biomedical enhancement. Often the scenarios portrayed by the media are science fictional, and as such will not be discussed in this work, where I am interested in an empirically grounded discussion of existing or highly plausible enhancement technologies, with a focus on genetic technologies. As pointed out by Atry in the context of genetic technologies aimed at athletic performance (Atry 2012), I think it is the bioethicists' responsibility to discuss real-world scenarios or scenarios which are at least plausible in the future, and that it is also the bioethicists' responsibility to avoid creating "media-like hype" around biomedical technologies, jeopardizing the ethical debate surrounding the same technologies. Borrowing a felicitous expression from American storyteller Raymond Carver,[1] we need to understand what we talk about when we talk about "enhancement."

The term "enhancement" as we refer to it in bioethics has its origin in genetic technologies in the late 1980s, when it arose in opposition to the term 'therapy' in the discussion of cases that were considered legitimate for the applications of gene transfer, in contrast to applications of the same technologies which were considered illegitimate and ethically troublesome. The first "gene therapy" trials involved the treatment of severe adenosine deaminase (ADA) immunodeficiency in 1990 at the US National Health Institutes. (Aiuti et al. 2009) Also known as "children in a bubble" disease, ADA is a devastating condition caused by a mutation in the ADA gene, which reduces or eliminates completely the activity of the corresponding enzyme, resulting in toxic levels of the same that lead to the death of lymphocytes (white blood cells). As a consequence, individuals affected lack virtually all immune protection and are prone to frequent and persistent opportunistic infections that can be life threatening. ("Adenosine Deaminase Deficiency" 2013) In the past thirty years, a series of clinical trials, employing different (and safer) vectors have been conducted. In particular, three recent studies have demonstrated that gene therapy can successfully correct the disease at the molecular level, and lead children to live a healthy life "out the bubble" to which they had been confined in the past. (Aiuti et al. 2009; Gaspar 2012)

At the time of the first clinical trials, the use of gene transfer to treat this severe immunological disease was seen as a morally justifiable means, even though risks for the individuals were very high, because of the severity of the disease and of the absence of alternative treatments. In parallel though, people started worrying about the prospect of other uses of gene transfer techniques, which would put subjects at a high risk without the same justification as the treatment of a life-threatening condition as ADA. Therefore, it

---

1   Raymond Carver, *What we talk about when we talk about love*, 1981

was initially thought that a terminological distinction (therapy/enhancement) could also serve as a moral distinction. (Elliott 2009) Things would not prove to be so easy, as we will see below.

In what follows, I adopt the framework developed by Menuz and co-authors who classify definitions of enhancements into four main categories: the implicit approach, the therapy-enhancement distinction, the improvement of general human capacities and the increase of well-being. (Menuz, Hurlimann, and Godard 2011)

The implicit approach

Authors who adopt an implicit approach would start discussing the ethical permissibility of a biomedical technology that they refer to as "enhancement technology" without spelling out what they mean with the word "enhancement". Some examples of this method can be found in (Mansour and Azzazy 2009; McKanna and Toriello 2010; Sadler 2010), among others. For example, Sadler, discussing the implications of enhancement technologies, while providing a critique of different accounts of the concepts of "dignity" as used in the transhumanist debate, takes for granted that the technologies he discusses can be classified as enhancements. (Sadler 2010) Two obvious shortcomings with such an approach are the following: (1) that it does not acknowledge the complexity of the "enhancement" concept, by assuming that all the people involved in the discussion are on the same page when referring to "enhancement," which is usually not the case; (2) that it does not acknowledge the constant evolution of social and political values, and therefore does not address the question of if, and when we can stop considering a technology as an enhancement. For these reasons an explicit approach to defining "enhancement" should be preferred. Of course, to be fair to Sadler and other authors who use an implicit approach, one cannot recapitulate the entire story of humankind – so to say – every time one writes, but one could, and should, make clear at the beginning of the text what definition of enhancement one is endorsing. Without doing so, it becomes impossible to discuss or bring forward the debate, as the different participants in the debate may be talking about different things.

Improvement of some human capacities/abilities

According to this widely used approach (Bostrom, Nick and Sandberg, Anders 2007; Allhoff, Lin, and Steinberg 2010; Harris 2007; Chan and Harris 2008), human enhancement is defined as the application of a technology 'to individuals so as to improve their body, mind or any ability beyond the species-typical level or statistically-normal range of functioning of a human being." (Menuz, Hurlimann, and Godard 2011)

For example, John Harris, one of the most prominent representatives of this approach, defines enhancement as "an improvement on what went before." (Harris 2007) He also adds: "If it wasn't good for you, it wouldn't be enhancement." (Harris 2007) Bostrom and Sandberg (2007) define enhancement as either a functional improvement over a "normal healthy state," or as the addition of a capacity that was not present in the human species at a former time point. This latter meaning of the term enhancement is then considered by Bostrom and Sandberg as they see enhancements as a means to transcend humanity as we know it today, and to produce better specimens of 'transhumans." Here is their definition:

> We define an enhancement as an intervention that causes either an improve-
> ment in the functioning of some subsystem (e.g. long-term memory) beyond
> its normal healthy state in some individual or the addition of a new capacity
> (e.g. magnetic sense). (Bostrom, Nick and Sandberg, Anders 2007, 3)

Note that, according to this definition, an enhancement is not necessarily a good thing, in contrast to John Harris' account (Harris considers the benefits of an enhancement technology only in relation to the individual, and not to society). Bostrom and Sandberg's definition is neutral in values. Improving on a human trait, or providing a new trait does not necessarily have positive effects on a person's life, as pointed out by De Melo-Martin in the welfaristic approach described below.

Increase in individual's wellbeing

This approach, which is adopted by a minority of scholars in the enhancement literature, defines enhancement as an increase on individual's wellbeing, or welfare. One well-known proponent of this value-laden account is Julian Savulescu:

> The term human enhancement is itself ambiguous. It might mean enhancement of functioning as a member of the species homo sapiens. This would be a functionalist definition. But when we are considering human enhancement, we are considering improvement of the person's life. The improvement is some change in state of the person – biological or psychological – which is good. Which changes are good depends on the value we are seeking to promote or maximize. In the context of human enhancement, the value in question is the goodness of a person's life, that is, his/her wellbeing. (Savulescu 2006, 324)

Therefore, Savulescu proposes a "welfarist" account of human enhancement, where the enhanced state is defined as a "capability" and a capability is "Any state of a person's biology or psychology which increases the chance of leading a good life … ." (2006, 324) (Note that the opposite of a capability is, in Savulescu's account, a disability, which is seen as a condition that diminishes the chances of an individual to lead a good life). While this approach has the advantage of sidestepping the problem of determining what "health" and "disease" are, and of determining a species-typical level, it does not solve the problem but merely relocates it, since this approach is also based on other controversial concepts, namely: human flourishing, wellbeing, welfare, etc. Moreover, this approach runs the risk of underestimating the social and cultural pressures that influence individual choices in life (see 2.1 for a discussion). It seems to me that Savulescu's definition of enhancement would more appropriately be referred to as "enhancement of wellbeing," which is a narrower class within all enhancements. Quite ironically, Saveluscu himself seems to recognize that the term enhancement is probably not the right one in his account. Writes Savulescu: "Enhancement is a *misnomer.* [emphasis added] It suggests luxury. But enhancement is no luxury. Insofar as it promotes wellbeing, it is the very essence of what is necessary for a good human life." (Savulescu 2009) As already noted, this absolutely positive connotation of the term "enhancement" is problematic, as the various applications of biomedical technologies need to be spelled out and discussed contextually before they can be univocally classified as positive, starting from an accurate description of the underlying science, and of their context of application. Not necessarily, and not in all contexts, enhancements will turn out to be good for the individual, or for society. As a matter of fact, the welfaristic approach does not take into consideration the social and collective consequences of the technology, but only the consequences of the technology on the individual's wellbeing.

The work by Inmaculada de Melo-Martin provides another example of a scholar who adopts a welfaristic approach to enhancement. In her work, de Melo-Martin objects to a "value-neutral" definition of enhancement. Her critique is based on the need to discuss what counts as a risk, and what counts as a benefit before entering the analysis of the risk/benefit ratio of the technology, and therefore the analysis of the value of an enhancement technology. (de Melo-Martin 2010) De Melo-Martin discusses also the necessity to spell out the different values underlying the application of a particular enhancement technology. For example, de Melo-Martin writes that some enhanced capacities, e.g. the ability to read a book in a very short time, or enhanced numerical abilities, should not necessarily be considered enhancements, as they are not necessarily related to a more fulfilled life, or to an enhanced wellbeing of the individual. (de Melo-Martin 2010) In this sense, an improvement on the human capacity for reading, or on human mnemonic skills for example, would not necessarily constitute an enhancement, unless we had decided *a priori* that such increases in human capacities were good things *per se*, on the basis of an intrinsic value – for example – in being able to read very fast.

The therapy-enhancement distinction approach

Finally, in this widely used approach (Daniels 2000; Resnik 2000; Wolpe 2002; President's Council on Bioethics (U.S.) 2003) human enhancement is defined through its goal and the condition or state (i.e., "disease" versus "health") that it aims to modify. This approach suggests that the "therapy/enhancement" distinction can function to draw a moral boundary between ethically permissible and ethically impermissible technologies (as it was also thought when the term "gene therapy" was coined, as illustrated before). In order to be valid, such an approach needs to be based on a clear definition of "health" and "disease," both concepts which are a source of considerable controversy. In addition, through such an approach interventions aimed at prevention and traditionally considered part of the scope of medicine (such as vaccination) should be viewed as enhancement. As I explain in the next section, I find this approach only of limited usefulness, due to the inherent problematicity of the therapy/enhancement distinction itself. Nevertheless this approach can still have a limited though useful role in the enhancement debate, as also illustrated below.

1.2 On the therapy versus enhancement distinction

As we have seen above, the term "enhancement" itself was coined in opposition to the term "therapy" in the context of gene transfer technologies. Consequently the analysis of this opposition is a necessary premise to understand the debate about enhancement technologies. The distinction was initially thought to possess an intrinsic moral significance, and to be able to demarcate ethically legitimate applications of gene transfer technologies from other not so legitimate applications. But it would not prove to be so easy. In this section I discuss the meaning and moral significance of the therapy/enhancement (T/E) distinction and the role it can play in the enhancement debate.

Norman Daniels spells out a limited defence of the T/E distinction. A US-based scholar, Daniels acknowledges that often this distinction is invoked in his country to demarcate conditions for which an insurance reimbursement would be appropriate (would-be treatments) and for conditions for which it would not (would-be enhancements). Such an approach could be generalised to include countries with a public health system or a mixed public-private health system between medical services for which the patient has to pay (even if partially), and services for which the patient does not have to pay. Writes Daniels:

> The treatment-enhancement distinction draws a line between services or interventions meant to prevent or cure (or otherwise ameliorate) conditions

that we view as diseases or disabilities and interventions that improve a condition that we view as a normal function or feature of members of our species. The line drawn here is widely appealed to in medical practice and medical insurance contexts, as well as in our everyday thinking about the medical services we do and should assist people in obtaining. (Daniels 2000, 309)

In this sense, the distinction is therefore closely related to the concept of "medical necessity" that is used in legislation in the US and Canada. (Hurley et al. 1997) Daniels offers the examples of children with a short stature receiving or not reimbursement for growth hormone (GH) therapy on the basis of the different underpinning causes of their short statures (only those children with a genetically identified cause would receive growth hormone therapy). Daniels raises the question whether such a differential reimbursement is justified, on the basis of the T/E distinction that forces us to treat "relevantly similar cases" in dissimilar ways. According to Daniels, providing treatment and reimbursement to a child, with short stature because of a genetic cause, and not providing treatment (or not reimbursing) to another child, who is short either because of idiopathic conditions, or only because he "feels short" in society, is unfair.

An excursion into the history of GH can be enlightening to better understand how the ethical dilemma of the scarcity of GH and the application of a scarce hormone have been justified in our recent past, in an occurrence of a problem that is still present today in many other instantiations. In the US in the 1950s, "stunted growth" was the term used to refer to "short stature," while "pituitary dwarfs" was the term used to refer to individuals deficient in the GH, and "primordial dwarves" to individuals affected by achondroplasia. (Rothman and Rothman 2003) In the '50s the only way to obtain GH (at that time known as "somatotropin") was to collect it from the pituitary glands of human cadavers. To overcome this scarcity, the US National Institutes of Health set up the National Pituitary Agency (NPA) at Johns Hopkins University in Baltimore to appeal for organ donation. (Rothman and Rothman 2003) How did the discourse surrounding the T/E distinction play out to decide how to allocate a scarce resource? Initially, GH was allocated only to "pituitary dwarfs," but vocal patient advocacy requests pressed the NIH to allocate it also to other individuals affected by stunted growth, independently of the genetic causes of the short stature. Note that it was never demonstrated that the administration of GH in individuals who had no GH deficiency was successful in the long-term to obtain an increase in stature, although it was demonstrated that they were able to cause spurts in growth in the short term. (Rothman and Rothman 2003)

In 1985, the problem of the scarcity of the resource was solved when the San Francisco Bay area biotech company Genentech started the synthetic production of GH (hence, the legal dispute with the University of California, San Francisco (UCSF) about the primacy of the invention, that was settled with $200M from Genentech to UCSF in 1999 (Barinaga 1999)). The discussion of the ethical use of the hormone was quenched by its new availability, but not extinguished, as a lingering one remained on to what extent patients' requests should be satisfied: what was, if any, the threshold under which an individual was to be classified as "short"? In 1990, after many decades of use, the NIH set up a clinical trial aimed at testing once and for all the efficacy of GH for short, non-hormone deficient children. (Tauer 1994) The results of the study, though, were not able to provide a clear-cut answer to the question because of the way it had been designed (Rothman and Rothman 2003) and the trial concluded that if a "condition" (e.g. short stature) caused "unhappiness, psychological pain, and social disadvantage," then interventions to remedy it should be considered "cures," irrespective of the biological cause. (Rothman and Rothman 2003)

As put by Daniels,

> It is not because there is something biologically distinctive about Johnny's condition, as opposed to Billy's, that has led us to describe Johnny as having a disease and Billy not. Rather, our "social construction" of disease draws on a set of values that happens to have singled out Johnny rather than Billy in this way. … Pointing to the line between treatment and enhancement is not, then, pointing to a biologically drawn line but is an indirect way of referring to valuations we make. (Daniels 2000, 313)

Finally, in July 2003, the FDA accepted the NIH recommendation and approved GH for "otherwise medically normal but unusually short" children. (LATimes Associated Press 2003) As pioneer US plastic surgeon Max Thorek was reported saying in the 1930s, anything that could raise "the quotient of patient happiness" was to be considered a legitimate medical task. (Rothman and Rothman 2003, 143) Hence, we could say that the conclusions of the NIH trial and FDA recommendation in 2003 represent an example of how the NIH constructed the category of "short stature" in order to respond to, and accommodate, patients' and society's requests.

Returning to the T/E distinction, what can we say about its significance, after we have argued that it is unfair to use it to demarcate "medical necessity" from "non-medical" necessity?

As have seen in this section, the use of the T/E distinction as a demarcation line between what is reimbursable and what is not reimbursable is problematic both from an historical and philosophical point of view. Daniels has also objected to the notion that the natural baseline of the T/E distinction, according to which disease and disability are departures from species-typical functioning, has an ontological importance. Even though I agree with Daniels that the distinction does not hold an ontological value, practically it has become a "focal point for convergence in our public conception of what we owe each other by way of medical assistance or healthcare protection" (Daniels 2000, 318), at least in North America. As such, there is a "primary rationale for including medical services in a healthcare benefit package" (Daniels 2000, 319) on the basis of this distinction. We can then conclude that, from a practical point of view, the T/E distinction can play a *prima facie* role in demarcating the scope of medical necessity from other scopes. This *prima facie* role though needs to withhold scrutiny and may not constitute a sufficient reason to treat similar cases (e.g. short children) in dissimilar ways.

While the distinction traced by Daniels is an interesting one and illustrates one of the concrete applications of labelling a technology as an "enhancement" or as "therapy," it is not one of the central concerns of this work focused mostly on genetic technologies. A more helpful perspective for the kind of contextual analysis and the choice of technologies that I carry out in this work is offered by David Resnik in relation to genetic technologies (2000), to whom I turn to conclude this section.

Genetic interventions are of particular interest for the scope of this work, which includes analysis of how they can be applied to enhance athletic performance in a professional sports context (sections 3.1 and 3.2), to decide what kind of children to bring into the world (sections 2.4 and 2.5) and to scout out children's talents (section 3.3). Resnik (2000) argues that the T/E distinction does not mark a firm boundary between ethical and unethical genetic interventions, for which it was originally conceived:

> Perhaps the most popular way of thinking about the moral significance of the therapy-enhancement distinction is to argue that the aim of genetic therapy is to treat human diseases while the aim of genetic enhancement is to perform other kinds of interventions, such as altering or "improving" the human body. Since genetic therapy serves morally legitimate goals, genetic therapy is morally acceptable; but since genetic enhancement serves morally questionable or illicit goals, genetic enhancement is not morally acceptable. (Resnik 2000, 366)

According to Resnik, this way of thinking of medical genetics is flawed as it based on at least two questionable assumptions, namely: (a) that we have a clear and uncontroversial account of health and disease (and we do not); and (b) that the goal of treating diseases is morally legitimate, while other goals are not. I concur with Resnik's analysis, but would also like to add that even if we were able to provide uncontroversial accounts of health and disease, it would not follow from this that using biomedical technologies for therapy purposes would be ethically justifiable, while the use of biomedical technologies for enhancement purposes would not. I am sympathetic with Resnik when he writes that what is really ethically troubling with the use of, for example, steroids by athletes, is not the non-medical use of steroid (or another pharmacological enhancer), but the violation of a value intrinsic to the context of professional sport. (Resnik 2000) In a paper co-authored with Mike McNamee and included in a slightly revised version in this work in section 3.2, we reach conclusions regarding the ethical permissibility of the same technology (gene transfer to raise the tolerance to pain) in two different contexts by spelling out the values intrinsic in the two contexts/practices. It is on the basis of this discussion at the level of values that we argue that the same technology could be ethically justified in one scenario and not in the other, not on the basis of the fact that it would count as a non-medical use of medicine.

Finally, another brief historical excursus could be useful to debunk the arguments that the use of biomedical technologies to enhance human capacities falls outside the scope of medicine, as it is argued by some scholars. The US pioneer surgeon, Max Thorek, provides a case in point. Already in the early 1900s Thorek was performing "therapeutical gonadal implantations," (i.e., testicular transplants collected mostly from apes and monkeys, but also from human cadavers) with the aim of elevating the level of male hormones (and supposedly, their sexual function) in the recipients, mostly older patients. (Rothman and Rothman 2003, 142–44) Between 1912 and 1923, Thorek performed more than one hundred testicular transplants at the American hospital in Chicago. Thorek was also among the first surgeons to perform breast reduction and abdominal excisions (the antecedents of contemporary plastic surgery practices), and in 1942 he wrote one of the first textbooks on plastic surgery. As a doctor, Thorek is a particularly interesting figure as his arguments could be seen as anticipating some of the arguments used today in support of pharmacological enhancement. Thorek was also a convinced champion of the legitimacy of enhancement within the scope of medicine, as he was convinced that "raising the quotient of patient happiness" was a legitimate medical task to pursue within the purview of the doctor's remittal. (Rothman and Rothman 2003, 142–44) The following quote exemplifies his thinking: "If the child can be given shapely ears he should have them for his own happiness; and who is to deny him that happiness if he can attain it?" (Rothman and Rothman 2003, 143), and also: "If surgery can restore happiness and enjoyment of life to an individual who has lost them, that is as strong a justification for its use as restoration to health." (Rothman and Rothman 2003, 143) Therefore, as it can be shown from this example and many others (for a more extensive analysis see: Scripko 2010), the arguments that enhancement technologies do not belong to the proper scope of doctor's profession are historically inaccurate.

1.3 Absolute versus positional goods

The last feature of the definition of "enhancement" that remains a matter of controversy and that I am going to analyse in this work hinges on the distinction between absolute and positional goods. Objects that everybody can enjoy without risking that they lose their status of "goods" belong to the former category. Examples would be music and sunlight. To the latter category belong goods that only some individuals can enjoy before the objects lose their status of goods (e.g. height. Not everybody can be tall; there must be at least one short person around. Note that the definition itself of being "tall" and of other positional goods changes over time, hence the importance of the discussion of enhancement in the context of society where they are found, as the same technology may count as an enhancement in one society but not in another). Goods that belong to this latter category are referred to as "positional goods" exactly as they place the individual who enjoys them in a better *position* with respect to another person. In other words, they offer a competitive advantage to the individuals.

Performance enhancing drugs in sport are one of the classical examples of instruments which provide a positional good, such as strength, endurance, resistance to pain, etc. Athletes seek to use performance enhancing drugs as they aim to obtain that competitive advantage which, even if marginally small, could secure them victory in competition. As I discuss in section 3.5 and more at length in (Camporesi and McNamee 2014), it is highly problematic that the demonstration of the performance enhancing effects of substances included in the World Anti-Doping Agency (WADA) Prohibited List is not a necessary criterion for inclusion in the List, but that only the potential to do so is sufficient (in combinatin with one of two criteria: potential risk to the athlete's health and the violation of the spirit of sport) for inclusion of a substance in the List. (WADA Code 2009)

John Harris views enhancements as absolute rather than positional good. He writes: "I defend them because they are good for people not because they confer advantages." (Harris 2007, 29) And elsewhere, he writes: "It follows [from the fact that something is good for people] that there can be nothing morally wrong with human enhancement per se." (Chan and Harris 2008) This view, while attractive in its simplicity, risks being too simplistic, as Harris neglects other important, and often fundamental factors, that underlie the reasons why individuals may seek enhancements. These factors are, more often than not, rooted in the search for a positional advantage, in the pressure of peers, of society, of the market, or in a combination of these factors. Note that these are the very same factors that result in social inequalities of access to enhancements. The problem of differential access to enhancement technologies is one of the most pressing ethical issues opened up by the new technologies. John Harris, by stating that an enhancement is always "good for people" (understood as the individual), is neglecting this fundamental issue of social inequalities. Indeed, not all things that on a subjective account can considered good for the individual are good also for society, nor are all things that can be considered on a subjective account "good for people" allowed in society (think of gambling, or of recreational drugs).

There are other values to take into account when judging the permissibility of enhancement technologies, apart from the personal freedom to pursue one's goals in life, and the relations and implications of the pursuit of one's own goals in life, including enhancements, need to be put in perspective with the pursuit of others' goals in a society, and with social values such as equality, and fairness.

Finally, it must also be noted that in practice it is very difficult, if not impossible, for a single enhancement technology to possess only characteristics that would qualify it as an absolute good, or only characteristics that would qualify it as a positional good. As a matter of fact, most enhancement technologies possess a combination of the two characteristics (see also the point on "relative ends" in the following section). DeGrazia offers the example of a technology that would give a person a "sunnier disposition" (while it is not clear from his writing how the technology could achieve the result of giving a person a sunnier disposition; probably DeGrazia has in mind Paxil, the antidepressant mentioned earlier in his work):

> One might think that an enhancement that gave someone a sunnier disposition, making his life more enjoyable, would provide a major intrinsic benefit without conferring any positional goods. One might think again. For a sunnier disposition offers competitive advantages to politicians, salespersons, real estate agents, and others whose job performance is improved by extroversion and the expression of optimism. (DeGrazia 2012, 129)

The absolute value of a biomedical enhancement acquires therefore an instrumental, external value when put in the context of the workplace. Plausibly, this would be a very common occurrence for most (if not all) biomedical enhancements. In addition, DeGrazia notes how positional goods create concerns about coercion, fairness (of access to the technology), and possibly concerns about collective self-defeat: if everybody, or at least a substantial portion of the population, had access to positional enhancements, they would lose their character of conferring an advantage to others. These are all issues that need to be taken into account when assessing the ethical permissibility of an enhancement technology in a particular context, as I aim to do in the following chapters. Before moving on to the analysis of the ethical and social implications of particular technologies though, let us briefly review the arguments that have been put forward and against enhancement in the bioethical arena.

1.4 Arguments in favour and against enhancement

One of the frequently raised objections to biomedical enhancements is that they alter human nature. This is what sends "shivers" – borrowing the expression from Lewens (2009), quoted at the beginning of this chapter – down the spine of some of the most vehement opponents of biomedical enhancements, including Leon Kass (Kass 2002) (former Chair of the President's Council on Bioethics under President George W. Bush), Francis Fukuyama (Fukuyama 2003), and Juergen Habermas (Habermas 2003). These authors embrace what Allen Buchanan refers to as "normative essentialism": they believe it is possible to derive substantive moral rules from reflection on human nature. (Buchanan 2009)

Habermas argues that interventions aimed at modifying human nature will affect "the necessary presupposition for being-able-to-be-oneself and [affect] the fundamentally egalitarian nature of our interpersonal relationships." (Habermas 2003, 13) For Habermas, what is most unsettling in genetic interventions and other kinds of biomedical interventions aimed at shaping oneself or others is "the fact that the dividing line between the nature we are and the organic equipment we give ourselves is being blurred." (Habermas 2003, 22) This blurring, he continues, shifts the "line between chance and choice," and by doing so "affects the self-understanding of persons who act on moral grounds." (Habermas 2003, 28) Moreover, this blurring of the categories of the "nature we are" and the "organic equipment" we give ourselves might "change our ethical self-understanding as a species" and give rise to a "novel, curiously asymmetrical type of relationship between persons." (Habermas 2003, 42) The possible blurring of the categories is especially problematic for Habermas as it touches upon "a necessary condition for an autonomous conduct of life and a universalistic understanding of morality." (Habermas 2003, 48)

At the other end of the spectrum of the debate, we find scholars who are so excited about the prospect of biomedical enhancements that they get "frissons" – borrowing again from Lewens (2009) – down their spines. Examples include (Bostrom, Nick and Sandberg, Anders 2007; Harris and Chan 2008; Chan and Harris 2008; Savulescu 2009) among others. As we have seen above, John Harris is among the strongest proponents of enhancements *tout court*. According to Harris, "Enhancing human capacities is taken to be a self-evident good," and we have a moral duty to enhance ourselves, and our children. I have already explained why I think that such an indiscriminate positive connotation of enhancement is incorrect. Here I would like to show why the discourse being used by Harris and other proponents of enhancement to frame new technologies as the most recent instantiation of the human pursuit for progress is only partially accurate.

In Harris' view, enhancing human capacities must be seen as the pursuit of a linear progress without any apparent end, along the lines of the Olympic motto of *"citius, altius, fortius"* (swifter, higher, stronger). Harris dismisses worries about enhancement as being a function of unnecessary anxiety, or of a similarly unnecessary fear of hubris. Together with the pursuit of "a linear progress," Harris stresses the continuity between those kinds of enhancements that humans have resorted to in the past, and the new kinds of biomedical enhancements that are being developed today, thanks to the most recent advances in biotechnology and biomedicine. But, as Erik Parens correctly pointed out: "It would be a mistake to think that the new biotechnologies are just more of the same. We should give up the arguments that take the form, 'we've always done it.'" And, while "It is true that we have always sought enhancement ..., arguments from precedent glibly excuse us from thinking about how new means to achieve old ends make a moral difference." (Parens 1998, 13) I agree with Parens on this point: it is not the existence of other established practices in society that justified the emergence of new ones which can be "brought back" to the former ones. Quite on the contrary, I think that it is the emergence of the latter ones that makes us reflect on what has been going on up to now. Note that this is also the approach I adopt (Camporesi 2013) that is included in this work in a revised form as section 3.4, where I discuss the application of genetic technologies to scout out a child's talent, which are by some scholars justified on the basis of other older and already established child-rearing practices.

Carl Elliott also discusses how enhancement technologies offer us new means to achieve old ends. Elliott outlined five problems created by these new means, which I will discuss in turn, pointing out how they relate to the analyses carried out in this work. (Elliott 2009)

Cultural complicity

The problem of cultural complicity was first identified by Margaret Olivia Little, who acutely pointed out how the demand for certain technologies is construed by cultural forces that can be harmful to the individual engaging in those practices. (Little 1998) Some examples include cosmetic surgery to delete markers of ethnicity, in order to enhance conformity to accepted European standards, or cosmetic surgery for breast or anti-ageing for women. What Little sees as problematic in these practices is that "by giving in" to these cultural forces, and agreeing to have a surgery, the underlying problematic societal trends become reinforced, and the individual who engages in them becomes in turn culturally complicit with them. (Little 1998) Cultural complicity seems to go hand in hand with the contemporary widespread rhetoric of self-fulfilment and the pursuit of happiness. As described by Scripko, the pursuit of wellbeing permeates the daily lives of Americans and enhancement technologies are seen as a way to liberate one's considered "authentic self," in a narrative where "being well becomes being one's optimal self in the society in which a person lives." (Scripko 2010, 294). Erik Parens also writes on this point:

> Given that many of us Americans feel it is our duty to pursue self-fulfillment and happiness on the Weberian model, it would not be surprising if many of us came to feel it our duty to use any means possible to fulfill it – including taking drugs like Prozac. (Parens 1998, 12)

Partly for this reason, much of the work in this book is focused on the US system. I also find that many of the ethical issues related to enhancement technologies are first applied in the US context, where the regulatory system is more liberal, and then find in the UK and Europe. For example, direct-to-consumer (DTC) genetic tests to scout out children's talents, which I analyze in chapter 3, first occurred in the US, while potential customers are not limited to US citizens. The analysis of the ethical permissibility of choosing to have deaf children through preimplantation genetic diagnosis (section 2.4) is also based on real-world case studies based in the US.

Relative ends

The problem of relative ends was already introduced in section 1.3, when discussing the intertwining of the qualities of absolute and positional goods in the same biomedical technology. The fact is that enhancement technologies are mostly sought by individuals because they can confer a positional advantage, not because they are "intrinsically" good. In other words, individuals seek enhancement technologies with the hope of gaining a "competitive advantage." Elliott discusses this in relation to the use of performance-enhancing drugs in sports, but it can be applied also to cognitive enhancements, and in general to all biomedical technologies. I analyse the problem of relative ends in my discussion of the use of gene transfer technologies applied to raise one's own tolerance to pain in endurance races, in section 3.4.

The role of the market

The third problem identified by Elliott relates to the role of the market, in particular to the US widespread practice of advertising enhancement technologies online or on television through DTC advertising. This has been possible in the USA since 1997, when the FDA relaxed its restriction on DTC advertising for prescription drugs. In particular, this is especially prevalent for anti-depressant drugs, and more recently for DTC-genetic tests to predict children's talent (discussed in sections 3.3).

Authenticity and human nature

The problem of authenticity relates to the narratives of restoration to "authentic self" through antidepressants that individuals resort to. These kinds of "restitution narratives," as put by Elliott (2009), are very common for people who consume antidepressants. Elliott points out how "restitution" may not be the most appropriate term since the self to which individuals say they are aspiring to never existed before, but was only desired or wished for. Note that the same language of authenticity can also be used for opposite ends (even though less frequently) by individuals who claim that they do not feel like themselves anymore when on antidepressants. Erik Parens (2005) has written extensively on the idea of "authenticity" and the role it playes in the discussion of enhancement technologies. (Parens 2005) Parens argues that the idea of "authenticity" is at the centre, even if not explicitly, of the debate on enhancement. He defines it as follows:

> While the idea of authenticity has a complex history, the core of it is that we are authentic when we exhibit or are in possession of what is most our own: our own way of flourishing or being fulfilled. To be separated from what is most our own is to be in a state of alienation. (Parens 2005, 35)

According to Parens, the current polarization of the debate on enhancement harks back to the different understandings of authenticity that the opponents and supporters of enhancement take as implicit assumptions of their arguments. These different understandings grow out of what Parens refers to as two different ethical "frameworks," where by framework he means a "constellation of commitments that support and shape our responses to questions about, among many other things, new enhancement technologies." (Parens 2005) One framework revolves around the concept of "gratitude," while the other revolves around the concept of "creativity." Parens points out how in the academic debate scholars often shift from one framework to the other, without being explicit about the meaning of "authenticity" they refer to. As I already pointed out at the beginning of this chapter, it is particularly important to spell out the values underlying the arguments when discussing a particular technology, especially when moral judgments are used to inform policy.

Arguments against enhancements and rooted in concerns about threat to human nature must be distinguished in two sorts of concerns: a) the threat of surpassing (or crossing the boundaries of) human nature; and b) the threat of altering human nature. Francis Fukuyama is one of the most prominent scholars opposing enhancement technologies, on the basis of an essential notion of human nature that would be undermined by the application of such technologies. (Fukuyama 2003) This essentialist notion of human nature is problematic on several fronts, as pointed out by David DeGrazia and Allen Buchanan among others. While recognizing that there are "powerful theoretical and intuitive grounds for maintaining that certain kinds of things have essential features" (DeGrazia 2012, 79) ("humanity" being one of those), DeGrazia objects to the argument that there is a single characteristic that could be regarded as the basis for the special moral status possessed by human beings. In other words, it is a logical fallacy to assume that human nature must involve "essential" features, where an essential feature for a kind of thing is defined as a "feature that X necessarily has in order to be a member of that kind." (DeGrazia 2012, 80) Buchanan also debunks these arguments on other grounds: (a) that on all plausible accounts, human nature "contains bad as well as good characteristics and there is no reason to believe that in every case eliminating some of the bad characteristics would so imperil the good ones as to make the elimination of the bad impermissible"; and (b) that modifications of human nature will not affect our ability to make judgment about the good. (Buchanan 2009) I concur with the analyses by DeGrazia and Buchanan, as I do not think that biomedical interventions would change the way a person perceives herself more than other kinds of parental intervention early in life already shape the kind of person one is and perceives herself, (see also: Camporesi 2013) nor that human nature should be considered as the basis of the moral self-understanding of a person. I also do not think that genetic interventions, only by virtue of being genetic, are substantially different from other kinds of interventions and that as such they should deserve a special scrutiny (See: Kakuk 2008 for a full argument debunking the genetic exceptionalism perspective, and my co-authored paper: Camporesi and Maugeri 2011 for a critical discussion of the exceptionalist perspective of the "Beyond Therapy" Report by the former President Council of Bioethics (President's Council on Bioethics (U.S.) 2003).

A Catch-22?

The final problematic issue of the enhancement debate identified by Elliott (2009) is exemplified by the following argument: enhancement technologies will in any case be pursued "somewhere else" in the world, once the technologies that enable them are developed, notwithstanding their moral justification. Consequently, as noted by Nicholas Agar, discussions on the ethical permissibility of enhancement technologies run the risk of falling prey to "technological determinism" about morality, defined as the certainty that "moral pronouncements have little or no influence on which technologies will be developed and who will use them." (Agar 2008, 170) Examples of technological determinism abound, as there will always be the possibility that some researcher "somewhere else" in the world, where regulation is more lax, could put in place and implement the biomedical technologies. Think for example of the claims, then revealed spurious, made by Panos Zavos and Severino Antinori in the early 2000s about reproductive cloning being achieved in Cyprus (Camporesi and Bortolotti 2008). Another example is China, where the regulation for gene therapy are more lax than in the US or Europe, and where gene therapy products have been approved that have been not elsewhere. (Wilson 2005) Many more examples can be found in (Meghani 2011; Cohen 2012), who discuss the migratory fluxes of medical and reproductive tourism and their multifaceted ethical and social implications.

It would therefore seem that we are left with a kind of "biotechnological catch-22," borrowing from Joseph Heller[2]: on the one hand, if we deliberate that research on the latest development of biomedicine is ethically impermissible, it would seem plausible to speculate that somebody else in another part of the world will still develop it, irrespective of our deliberation. If that were the case, we will be left with the not easy question of what to do with the products of knowledge developed elsewhere with means that we have deemed ethically impermissible (for example, the results of clinical trials developed without a proper informed consent in developing countries, or on prisoners, or on other ethically problematic situations etc.). On the other hand, we could

---

2   Joseph Heller, *Catch 22*, 1961.

recognize the fact that somebody else, elsewhere in the world, will develop the technology, and we could renounce deliberating in this field of morality.

That the latter choice would be a very dangerous move since a consistent application of this reasoning would lead to a retreat on morality on many different fronts. To escape this biotechnological catch-22, we must recognize, with Agar, that "technological determinism does not render morality redundant. There will almost certainly never be a human society in which there is no murder – but this is no reason not to pass moral judgements on murderers." (Agar 2008, 172)

Having concluded that a philosophical analysis of enhancement technologies (and therefore, this work!) is not completely useless, I will now proceed to the contextual analysis of case studies. In the next chapter I turn to the consideration of arguments against genetic technologies aimed at enhancing individuals and future generations, analysing first the arguments based on parallelisms with the old eugenics, and then proceeding to consider the application of genetic technologies to choose what kind of children to bring into the world.

Chapter 2

From bench to bedside: Genetic technologies to choose children's traits

2.1 Genetic enhancements and the ghost of eugenics

Arguments against enhancement often single out genetic technologies as being especially unacceptable from a moral point of view. Both pre-implantation diagnosis (PGD) and other genetic techniques aimed at human enhancement, along with screening programs to detect genetic disorders, have prompted a fierce controversy about the resurgence of eugenics. The recent writing by Gina Maranto exemplifies this current trend:

> The unfortunate truth is that discredited ideas never do die, they just rise again in slightly altered forms – witness eugenics. Despite the horrors perpetuated in its name, including forced sterilization and the Holocaust, the eugenic impulse is with us still. One of the forms it takes is schemes for "improving" offspring through the selection and manipulation of embryos. (Maranto 2013)

In the first part of this chapter I shall address the question of whether such parallelisms between the Holocaust, old eugenics and contemporary modes of improving ourselves and others through genetic technologies are indeed justified. Before discussing whether contemporary modes of genetic interventions can be classified as eugenics, and what if anything is wrong with that, it is necessary though to take a step back to understand what we talk about when we talk about "eugenics," borrowing again from Raymond Carver. In order to do that, I will provide a brief comparative historical overview of eugenics in the

UK, the US and Scandinavia, dividing the analysis into the periods: a) "classical eugenics" (1883-1945), b) "modern eugenics," from the end of WWII to the first "test tube baby" (1946-1978), and c) "contemporary eugenics," from the birth of Louise Brown until now (1978-2014). I will highlight similarities and differences between the three periods and address whether the objections to classical and modern eugenics are still valid today.

Classical eugenics: 1883-1945

I refer to "classical eugenics" as the first period, spanning from the invention of the word in 1883 by Francis Galton to the end of the WWII. The word "eugenics" comes from Greek, meaning "good in birth." As the story goes, after reading Charles Darwin's *The Origin of Species*, Galton concluded that much human misery was caused by physical problems that were passed down through generations. Galton thought that such misfortunes could be avoided through positive measures aimed at actively encouraging reproduction among the "fittest," and actively discouraging reproduction among the less fit. On May 16, 1904 Galton delivered a lecture on the definition, scope and aims of eugenics before the British Sociological Society at a meeting held at the School of Economics and Political Science in London (currently the London School of Economics). While Galton defined eugenics in positive terms as "the science which deals with all influences that improve the inborn qualities of a race; also with those that develop them to the utmost advantage,"(Galton 1906, 35) he did not necessarily exclude negative measures in the interest of the State and the British race. At that time, fear of "race degeneration" and of the decline of the British Empire from the international scene were pervasive.

Indeed, Galton considered efforts aimed at improving race a duty both for the individual and the society. He wrote, "An enthusiasm to improve the race is so noble in its aim that it might well give rise to the sense of a religious obligation." (Galton 1906, 25) He also thought that the means justified the end, as he wrote: "We are justified in following every path in a resolute and hopeful spirit that seems to lead towards that end." (Galton 1906, 33) For Galton, eugenics was to become a new, "orthodox religion," as he was persuaded that "few things are more needed by us in England than a revision of our religion, to adapt it to the intelligence and needs of the present time." (Galton 1906, 59) The creed of eugenics for Galton was founded upon an active idea of human evolution towards the "fittest race." In this regard, his assumptions are not that different from those contemporary scholars who view biomedical enhancements as a means to evolve the human species. (John Harris 2007; A. Buchanan 2011) Wrote Galton more than one hundred years ago: "Evolution … assumes an infinitely more interesting aspect under the knowledge that the intelligent action of the human will is, in some small measure, capable of guiding its course." (Galton 1906, 69) Writes John Harris today: "This 'progress of evolution' is unlikely now to be achieved accidentally or by letting nature take its course. If illness and poverty are indeed to become rare misfortunes, this is unlikely to occur by chance. … It may be that a nudge or two is needed: nudges that will start the process … of replacing natural selection with deliberate selection, Darwinian evolution with 'enhancement evolution'." (Harris 2007, 11)

Galton developed a biometric model of heredity that he thought could be "harnessed to a social programme for improving the human breed through selective mating." (Porter 2011, 272) As said above, "selective mating" included both positive and negative measures to prohibit the less fit from breeding, and as pointed out by Dorothy Porter (2011), the combination of degenerationist fears about the decline of the British race, and the fear of Britain's imperial decline, were the two main movers of the eugenics movement in the UK, which aimed at reversing the degenerative trends. (Porter 2011) The Victorian poor were considered a "race apart," and described as "noticeably smaller, stunted, scrawny, potbellied, rickety, scarred by sores, scrofulous lumps, and other stigmata of sickness." (Porter 2011, 220) An Interdepartmental Committee was set up in England to investigate the question of physical deterioration, and in 1904 produced a report reaching the main conclusion that physical deterioration was due to bad environment and unsuitable nutrition, and not to biological causes of the degeneration of race. Notwithstanding the conclusions of the 1904 report, the fear of racial degeneration continued to propel eugenics policies in England. In 1907, the British "Eugenics Education Society" was founded, with declared both positive and negative aims: to "protect the unborn" through selective breeding, to perform "voluntary sterilization" on the lower classes and to "sequestrate the unfit." In the UK, negative eugenics measures targeted mainly the feeble-minded with sterilisation or life-long detention (sequestration) upon certificates by two doctors. This was made possible after the enactment of the Mental Deficiency Act in 1913. To note also that a bill introduced by Winston Churchill advocating compulsory sterilisation of the "feeble minded and insane classes" was only narrowly defeated in 1913. (Porter 2011) After this failed attempt, England was never to pass laws restricting marriage among the "feeble-minded" nor compelled their sterilisation.

Contrary to what happened in England, forced sterilisation laws were passed in over thirty states in the US before 1914, the first being Indiana in 1907. (Lombardo 2011) In the US, fear of "degeneration" focused on immigrants from Eastern and Southern Europe, as well as non-whites. The Model Eugenical Sterilization Law, published by the US Eugenics Record Office in 1914, provided for the sterilisation of quite a large category of individuals including the "feeble-minded, insane, criminalistic, epileptic, inebriate, diseased, blind, deaf, deformed, and dependent." (Lombardo 2011) Then in the 1920s the ideas stemming from Mendel's genetics came into fashion, and with them came a long list of ill-defined traits, collected under the category of "feeble-mindedness." This in practice became a "catch-all category linked more closely to poverty and perceived anti-social behaviour than to organic mental deficiency" (Dorr 2011, 164). Again as pointed out by Dorothy Porter, in the US eugenics was "moulded by racialist concerns with immigration restriction" (Porter 2011, 273), and its principles were incorporated in the Immigration Restriction Act of 1924, which set quotas limiting the immigration of "biologically inferior" ethnic groups into the United States (South and East Europe) and favoured the entrance of Northern Europeans. (Suter 2007, 907) In 1908 the American psychologist Henry H. Goddard introduced the I.Q. test, which then became the main barrier for immigration at Ellis Island.[1] Keeping "unfit" immigrants from entering the US though was not considered a sufficient measure by eugenicists. Negative eugenics measures aimed at reducing or prohibiting the reproduction of the

---

1   For a powerful and historically accurate fictional representation, see also the 2006 movie "Golden Door" directed by Emanuele Crialese.

feeble-minded were also soon implemented. In the United States, Charles Davenport, who would become the leader of American eugenics, received funds to study evolution from the Rockefeller Society and develop therein a eugenics research facility, a testament to the close link between the two. The Rockefeller Society was to fund eugenics studies worldwide, including in Italy in the aftermath of the 2nd World War, as described in the next section. In 1909, Davenport became the Director of the Cold Spring Harbor laboratory on Long Island, where in 1910 he founded the Eugenics Record Office. (McCabe and McCabe 2011). Between 1968 and 1972, the US witnessed a sterilisation explosion: approximately 2 million Americans underwent sterilisation in 1973 alone (!) (Dorr 2011, 175) Often the sterilisations were performed under the guise of other abdominal surgeries on unaware patients, in what became known as "Mississippi appendectomies." (Roberts 2000)

In a similar fashion to what happened in the UK, the US definition of "fitness" and "unfitness," and consequently the targets for sterilisation, corresponded to American's white Protestant racial class prejudices (the contemporary "WASP," or "White Anglo-Saxon Protestant" racial, political and religious ideal). Baby contests and "fitter families" contests were very popular up to the 1970s all over the US in state fairs, and some have persisted even up to today, as represented in the 2006 movie "Little Miss Sunshine" directed by Dayton and Faris, and in the TV series "Toddlers & Tiaras." (Dorr and Logan 2011, 70–71)

Note also that in the US, in the State of California, a recent report published by the Center for Investigative Reporting (CIR) uncovered the sterilisation of more than 50 female inmates from 2006 to 2010 without required state approvals. (Johnson 2013) The report made the headlines and stirred a fierce controversy about the resurgence of eugenics, which is still on-going. (Easley 2013; Ohlheiser 2013; Sullivan 2013)

Sweden and all of Scandinavia witnessed extensive sterilisation efforts just before WWI. These were prompted by eugenic policies that emerged together with the emergence of the social welfare state, which developed in Scandinavia in the 1930s and '40s. (Broberg and Roll-Hansen 2005) For this reason, the authors have coined the term "welfare state eugenics" for Sweden, Norway, Finland and Denmark, where eugenics policies were seen as a subclass of a broader "Hygiene Movement," precursor of the much praised North European model of the welfare state. (Broberg and Roll-Hansen 2005) The interests of the individual were to be subordinated to the interests of the state. At that time, as already pointed out for the US and the UK, there was a pervasive worry about "race degeneration," and the declining birth rate, which pushed forward the eugenic policies. In all of Scandinavia sterilisation was used mainly for the mentally retarded (elsewhere referred to as the "feeble-minded"), and to a lesser extent as a measure of social control towards alcoholics, criminals, and in general – along similar lines to what happened in the US – towards all those who were considered incapable of caring and raising children. This category was stretched to include the category of "exhausted mothers," or mothers who had too many children and were considered incapable of raising them/taking proper care of them. (Broberg and Roll-Hansen 2005)

Notably, there was very little public opposition, and in general very little if any debate about the passing of eugenic and sterilisation laws in Scandinavian countries. Contrary to what happened in Sweden, in Denmark, Norway and Finland, sterilisation remained on a "voluntary" basis, but even if direct coercion was not used, many other indirect means of coercing people to consent to sterilisation were used, including having sterilisation as a condition for leaving an institution, getting an abortion, or getting permission to marry. As already pointed out, these measures were not so distant from the sterilisation laws implemented in the US up to the 1970s. Also to note that there was no revision of the eugenics laws after WWII, and that the social democratic belief in eugenics continued up to the 1950s. In Sweden (the most 'efficient' of Scandinavian countries for the implementation of eugenic laws, with up to 60,000 people sterilised between 1935 and 1975) the Sterilization law were not abrogated until as recently as 1975. (Broberg and Roll-Hansen 2005) Eugenics policies and laws were also implemented in Italy, though they were aimed at a different ideal of individual, which incorporated Fascist and Catholic values in fertility and privileged quantity versus quality of offspring. (Cassata 2011)

It is also of interest to note that US eugenic laws, and not Germany laws as it might be thought, served as a model for the eugenic laws of Sweden and Norway. (Dorr 2011, 172) As already noted, Sweden had compulsory sterilisation and both in relative and absolute number it was the most efficient Scandinavian country at implementing sterilisation. The uniqueness of Scandinavian countries in this regard is that they were the only countries in

Europe (with the addition of Estonia) that introduced sterilisation laws in the 1930s under democracies. In Scandinavia, sterilisation was considered a rational and humane solution to the problem of economic and social burden of mentally retarded individuals. (Broberg and Roll-Hansen 2005) The welfare state helped many, but also demanded much from few.

Therefore, as this brief excursus shows, eugenics policies were the results of different ideological motivations and backgrounds in Scandinavia, Germany, UK, Italy, and the US. In England, eugenics policies focused more on "class" than on "race," and as pointed out by Dorothy Porter, eugenics was "less a scientific pursuit than a lay, voluntary movement of social reform in the Edwardian period." (Porter 2011, 250) Always in England, the "unfit" were defined within the conventional terms of Victorian-British reform movements, where the social status combined with the considered anti-social behaviour produced the "unfitness" that included many different categories of deviant behaviour (alcoholism, promiscuity, criminality ...) which were understood as hereditary traits and lumped together with other traits, such as mental retardation, considered to be "inborn errors of metabolism." (Porter 2011, 250-1) Note that this is not so different from the definition of the "unfit" in the US on the basis of the "WASP" model ("White Anglo-Saxon Protestant").

In Sweden, however, race biology became a subject of institutionalised scientific research before the WWI, and eugenics was considered a "philosophy" of social efficiency that fitted easily within a welfare ideology. Of the more than 60,000 sterilisations that were performed in Sweden between 1935 and 1975, over 90 % were performed on women, although it must be noted that these numbers do not distinguish the sterilisations that were performed as a measure of contraception for women who had no other means. Swedish proponents of eugenics were very vocal in stressing the difference of Swedish eugenic laws with German eugenic laws, claiming that in Sweden sterilisations were not compulsory except for the "legally incompetent." But, as noted above, other less coercive means were abundant, and sterilisation was a precondition for release from an institution, and for getting married.

As a matter of fact – and as exemplified in the quote by Maranto reported at the beginning of this chapter – it is the atrocities committed in Germany in the name of racial purity which gave the contemporary bad connotation to the word "eugenics." Such a view though is over-simplistic, as highlighted below.

Indeed, in the US before the war the term "eugenics" started being used in the broader acceptation of "good," not only "good in birth." As pointed out by Lombardo, the term "encompassed everything from proud pedigrees to healthy births" and over time the invocation of "eugenics" became so widespread that in 1915 a Chicago politician run for alderman as 'the eugenics candidate." (Lombardo 2011, 45)

After WWII the use of the word deliberately fell out of practice. But note though that even now in the US, only a handful of states have repealed their eugenics sterilisation laws, although the programs have been inactive for years in those states that still retain such legislation. (Suter 2007)

Modern eugenics: 1945-1978

I refer to "modern eugenics" as the period that goes from the end of WWII to the first "test tube-baby," Louise Brown, who was born in Oldham, England, on July 25, 1978. (BBC News Health 2013) In those thirty years the practice of genetic counselling was established. Initially, it was limited only to prenatal screening for a very limited number of genetic diseases that present an abnormal karyotype (i.e. number and form of chromosomes), such as Down syndrome and other trisomies. During this period, choices concerning the future genetic pool shifted from the State to the parents, whose aim in using genetic screening was to have children free from disabilities. The nascent practice of genetic counselling was seen as a way for prospective parents to exercise autonomy and reproductive freedom. There was no mention of race or the community's gene pool in the prospective parents' decisions, but in the great majority of cases there were parents who wanted to give their children the best chance in life possible. (Suter 2007) The parents' decision was exercised without coercion from the State, even though as noted by Suter some kind of social pressure aimed at avoiding severe disabilities was still present. (Suter 2007)

Italy played a prominent role in the international scene of medical genetics in the second post-war period, as it was chosen as the seat of the International Congress of Genetics in 1948. (Cassata 2011) This decision placed the Italian Society of Genetics and Eugenics (SIGE) in a prominent position in relation to the international scientific community. In Italy, as pointed out by Francesco

Cassata, applied medical genetics to the new practice of genetic counselling was generally presented – and received – as a worthy and modern form of eugenics. (Cassata 2011) In Italy, the spectre of Nazism did not obfuscate in the public's eyes the possibility of a good eugenics based on "irrefutable scientific knowledge, and above all, conducted with liberal, non coercive methods." (Cassata 2011, 304) Italian eugenics during the second World War indeed differentiated itself[2] from the Nordic measures of eugenics by encompassing a natalist approach to population policies supported by the Fascist regime. This approached favoured "quantity" versus "quality" of the Italian race, and supported the power of a "regenerative eugenics" through the values of fertility and prolificity in contrast to the "conservative eugenics" of Anglo-Saxons or Germans which aimed at the sterlisation or elimination of "defective" individuals. (Cassata 2011)

Milan became the new capital of eugenics after the second World War: the first Italian genetic counselling centre was established at the Milan State University in 1946, and two years later the first public, "municipal eugenic counselling centre" was also established at the Milan Policlinic. (Cassata 2011, 309) The two centres were working primarily with premarital counselling for thalassemia and other kinds of microcytic anaemia which are endemic in Italy, especially in Sardinia and in other isolated regions of the country, as healthy carriers (heterozygous for the mutation) had from an evolutionary standpoint an advantage by being more resistant to malaria than the homozygous individual. (Luzzatto 1981) In 1954, the Rockefeller Foundation already mentioned above financed research conducted by a group based in Rome and aimed at tackling "the eugenic aspect of the microcythemic problem, the establishment of official registers of persons carrying this gene, marriage counselling in some form." (Cassata 2011, 324) Even Pope Pius XII intervened, publicly advising in favour of the necessity of premarital counselling, but advising against marriage prohibition based on genetic incompatibilities, as genetics "could not regard the human being in the same way as any other animal and vegetable species," meaning that human beings had inviolable rights (including the right to marry, and to have children) that – and this was presumably the

---

2   SIGE officially withdrew its membership from the International Federation of Eugenic Organisations in 1932.

implicit comparison underlying the Pope's statement – Mendel's peas did not have. (Cassata 2011, 328, 342)

As correctly noted by Suter though, even if parental decisions in this second phase were "voluntary," they were still taking place within a normative context biased towards prophylaxis (Suter 2007, 923), and prospective parents could very well feel societal pressure regarding the use of genetic technologies:

> All of these factors – advancing technologies and cultural norms – may exert a coercive effect on individuals' reproductive choices. As the American Medical Association Council on Ethical and Judicial Affairs has stated, the most likely risk today is not "overt eugenics" or "government imposed constraints on marriage and reproduction" but instead that the aggregate result of individual choices creates societal and cultural norms which substantially influence or limit the scope of autonomous decision making in regard to the use of genetic technology. (Suter 2007, 936)

In general, though, it can be said with a reasonable degree of confidence that during this second phase genetic counselling strived toward an ideal of "non-directiveness," advising but not directing – keeping in mind the limits of this in practice – prospective parents. Moreover, the actions of the parents were always aimed at bringing into the world children free from disabilities. As we will see, this was going to change in the current era of eugenics, as the choice of which traits parents were able to screen for was also expanding, and with it the motivation of the parents for using genetic technologies for selective reproduction..

Contemporary eugenics: 1978 to now

This period in eugenics, beginning with the birth of the first test tube baby Louise Brown in 1978 and continuing to today can be considered as "contemporary eugenics," though in section 2.2 I will argue that a more appropriate term for this period would actually be "*eligogenics.*" This period comprises the use of various assisted reproduction techniques or AR techniques (such as in vitro fertilization or IVF, and intraplasmic sperm injection or ICSI) for couples having problems conceiving, and, from 1989 on, the possibility of pre-implantation genetic diagnosis (PGD) in certain countries, depending on regulations. The motivations behind the couples' decisions are initially similar to those present in the second period, but people now have many more tools to exercise their reproductive freedom and to choose what kind of children they want to bring into the world.

The year 1989 represented a landmark year not only for the fall of Berlin wall and the lifting of the Iron Curtain, but also because it was the year when the first babies who had been selected as free from a genetic condition using PGD were born. UK scientists Alan Handyside and Robert Winston used this technique to select embryos free from cystic fibrosis, adrenoleukodystrophy (a severe neurodegenerative disorder due to the accumulation of fatty acids in the neurons) or X-linked mental retardation. (Handyside et al. 1992)

PGD encompasses a series of different methods aimed at testing the embryo for genetic conditions, and it involves the removal of a single cell at the stage of blastomere from the 6 to 8-cell embryo stage using a fine glass needle to puncture the zona pellucida (i.e., coat) and aspirate the cell. (SenGupta and Delhanty 2012) As PGD is technically more challenging than IVF, it is estimated that only a couple of thousand babies around the world have been born following PGD, against an estimated more than 5 million children following IVF (up to 2012). (Harper et al. 2012) PGD is currently offered at only eight centres in the UK, all of which are fertility clinics licensed by the British Human Fertilization and Embryology Authority (HFEA). The list of the conditions available for screening for PGD is also constantly updated, and in 2012 it was altered to include only conditions deemed particularly severe. The entire list of licensed conditions for PGD can be found on the website of the HFEA and is periodically revised. (HFEA 2013)

PGD is prohibited in several countries, including Austria and Switzerland, and permitted with very strict limitations in Germany and Italy. (Soini 2007) In Germany, PGD was completed prohibited until recently, when on July 11, 2011, the Parliament passed a law allowing couples to resort to PGD to screen embryos only if the parents have a predisposition to a "serious genetic disease." All applications for PGD must pass an ethics panel and couples are required to undergo genetic counselling. The bill outlines an exception to the 1990 Embryo Protection Act that bans PGD and any embryo experimentation. The Act remains intact and recommends a three year jail term for anyone using an embryo in a way that fails to promote its survival. (Beier and Beckham 1991; Gottweis 2002) Previously, PGD was banned in Germany on "eugenic" grounds and many people went abroad (to Switzerland, the UK, and France, for example) on "medical tourism" trips, which are increasingly common especially for reproductive purposes within Europe. (Tuffs 2011; Zanini 2011) The more severe limitations to any kind of embryo manipulation or discard in Germany can and should be understood in their historical context as a moral and political response to the heinous crimes of the Holocaust.

In Italy, PGD has been prohibited since 2004, with the promulgation of law 40/2004, on different grounds from the German prohibition, but also to be understood historically due to the strong and persistent Vatican influence. (Fineschi, Neri, and Turillazzi 2005) In 2012, the European Court of Human Rights (ECHR) ruled the Italian law 40/2004 unconstitutional as it "violates the right to respect for private and family life" guaranteed by Article 8 of the European Convention on Human Rights. (White 2012) In addition, the judges noted the inconsistency of the Italian law, which "on one side deprives the applicants access to PGD and on the other authorizes them to perform therapeutic termination of pregnancy when the fetus is affected from this same disease." (White 2012; Turone 2012) The case was brought to the ECHR through the case of Rosetta Costa and Walter Pavan v. Italy (no. 54270/10). (ECHR 2012) Costa and Pavan are asymptomatic carriers of cystic fibrosis who were seeking AR techniques to conceive in vitro and PGD to select an embryo free of the cystic fibrosis mutation. The couple complained they were "forced to abort" their potentially disabled child in 2010, while had they been able to resort to PGD earlier on, abortion would not have been necessary. The ECHR awarded the couple €15,000 as compensation, but denied further complaints of discrimination. (White 2012) To note that, unlike a national court, the ECHR does not directly have the power to overturn Italian law, and the government has the right to appeal the decision, which the Italian government did under Prime Minister Biondi in November 2012.[3] (Maggiorelli 2012; Biondi 2013) As noted above, the Italian ban on PGD was part of a law on assisted reproduction, introduced in 2004, which ruled that assisted reproduc-

---

3   A decision on the appeal has not been reached at the time of finalizing this
    work (July 2014).

tion was only available to infertile heterosexual couples. (Fineschi, Neri, and Turillazzi 2005) The same law ruled that it was illegal to freeze or destroy human embryos or use donated sperm and eggs. This has led to a dramatic decrease in the rates of successful delivery following IVF (in vitro oocytes do not freeze as well as embryos and are not viable upon thawing) (Levi Setti et al. 2013) and to a dramatic increase in the flux of reproductive tourism from Italy to Spain, Switzerland and other more permissive countries in the EU. (Manna and Nardo 2005; Zanini 2011)

The US has a more permissive approach to PGD. As described by Mc-Cabe and McCabe (2011), in the US there are state-based regulatory authorities that establish the rules of medical practice conduct and misconduct. In addition to state-based regulation, corporate incentives and pharmaceutical lobbies have a strong influence on the regulation of AR and PGD clinics. (McCabe and McCabe 2011) What happens is that while in theory, clinics are allowed to provide PGD for any possible technical reason for which it is requested, in practice, clinicians in the US adhere to professional guidelines issued by the American Society for Reproductive Medicine.[4] (Practice Committee of the ASRM 2006)

In the last ten years, PGD has been used not only to avoid traits traditionally considered as "disabilities," but also to choose the sex of the child. The use of PGD to select babies of a particular sex for "family balancing reasons" (an expression very broadly applied also in cases where the couple seeking PGD has only one child, or has no child but has a preference to conceive a child of a determined sex) is permitted in the US, (Ethics Committee of the American Society of Reproductive Medicine 2004) whereas it is currently banned in the UK by the HFEA. The HFEA allows sex selection only to avoid passing of conditions that are X-linked, i.e. for which a girl, having two X chromosomes, would not manifest the disease but only be a carrier, whereas a boy would manifest the disease. (HFEA 2002; HFEA Act 2008) Many ethicists (see for example McCarthy 2001; Dahl 2004; Harris 2005; Wilkinson and Garrard 2013) and members of the public (Adam 2012; Connor 2013) have recently argued in favour of lifting the HFEA ban. I would not be surprised that the HFEA were to reconsider its decision and announce a new public

---

4   http://www.asrm.org/PGDSIG/ [accessed July 18, 2014]

consultation on the topic in the next couple of years or so.

As mentioned above, the period that I refer to as 'contemporary eugenics' differs from modern eugenics not only because the range of traits available for screening with PGD has been expanding, but also because the motivations of parents to use PGD have been expanding too. For example, in the US, PGD has been used to choose for traits traditionally considered a disability, such as deafness or achondroplasia (genetic dwarfism). A 2006 survey of 190 American PGD clinics found that 3% reported having intentionally administered PGD "to select an embryo for the presence of a disability." In section 2.3 of this chapter I analyse the case of choosing deafness with PGD.

2.2 Eugenics and *"Eligogenics"*: past and present objections

As we have seen, the aim of eugenics was the improvement of the overall quality of the gene pool, to be achieved both through positive and negative means. Reproduction was understood as an act with social consequences, not a private matter. The interests of the state always took precedence over the interests of the individuals, and there was little or no discussion about it. Direct and less direct means of coercion were used to restrain the mentally retarded, those considered feeble-minded and in general all those considered a burden to society from reproducing.

Are the ethical objections against classical eugenics still valid toward modern practices of reproductive genetic choices? The key question to address is whether eugenics was wrong in its very inception. Gina Maranto, quoted at the beginning of this chapter, argues that wrong ideas never die, but come back under a new guise. (Maranto 2013) But her statement needs qualifying. First of all: can the contemporary use of genetic technologies to choose to have deaf or dwarf children still be called "eugenic"? There is no word, yet, to define such practices. The only attempt to date is by Isabel Karpin, who in 2008 defined it as "negative enhancement." Such a definition, though, seems to carry a negative connotation which is foreign to the intentions of the parents, who consider deafness or dwarfism not to be disabilities, but "only "differences" that will enable their children to "enter into a rich, and shared culture." (Sanghavi 2006) As an alternative, Sonia Suter (2007) suggested the word "neo-eugenics" for all contemporary uses of genetic technologies to choose for selective reproduction. Writes Suter:

> I refer to these modern practices as "neoeugenics" to suggest that they share
> some key features with classic eugenics – e.g., the goal of increasing "good
> birth" – and that they differ because they occur primarily at the individual,
> rather than state, level. (Suter 2007, 898)

Therefore, in contemporary practices the locus of what is "good" has changed
from the level of the state to the level of the individual. For this reason, it
seems to me that another word that could better capture the full spectrum of
parental choices to also include choosing deafness and dwarfism may be "*eligogenics,*" where "eligo" comes from the Latin "eligere" or "to choose". It seems
to me that the term "eligogenics" better captures the narratives used by the
prospective parents when asked why they are resorting to PGD, i.e. they are
claiming to be "choosing" what is good for their children. In the rest of this
chapter I will refer to contemporary uses of genetic technologies to choose
traits for the offspring, including choosing traits traditionally considered disabilities, as eligogenics.

Buchanan and co-authors argue that, reprehensible as much of the eugenic program was, there is something unobjectionable and perhaps even morally
required in the part of its motivation that sought to endow future generations
with genes that might enable them to live better lives. The authors also argue
that these motivations need not to be abandoned, if they can be pursued just-
ly. (Buchanan et al. 2000, 27-60) Suter writes along similar lines, (referring to
contemporary eugenics practices as "neo-eugenics"):

> Neoeugenics (and even eugenics), I shall argue, is not per se problematic.
> That is, many of the underlying goals are legitimate. This is not to say that
> neoeugenics is not problematic in practice; … The analysis, however, is high-
> ly contextual, depending both on social factors and individual circumstances.
> (Suter 2007, 899)

I will now consider the objections to classical eugenics and discuss whether
they can be applied also to eligogenics practices, following the analysis by

Buchanan et al. (2000), who identify five possible answers to why eugenics was morally wrong. (Buchanan et al. 2000, 27–60)

Replacement

The first objection identified (replacement, not therapy) is one of the arguments often brought forward today by the disability rights movement scholars. (Parens and Asch 2000, 3-44) These scholars argue that the use of genetic technologies aimed at choosing "better people" is *de facto* devaluing disabled existing people, and also harming them as it takes away from them important resources to improve their conditions in society. This objection is often referred to as the "expressivist objection," which at its core claims that the use of PGD or termination of pregnancy expresses discriminatory attitudes towards disabled people. However, it is important to note that not all disability right scholars unavoidably see PGD or other attempts at preventing impairments (including termination of pregnancy) as necessarily sending negative messages about disabled people. According to Tom Shakespeare, for example, it is "not inconsistent to support the rights of existing disabled people, while seeking to prevent more people from becoming impaired." (Shakespeare 2013, 120) What is important, adds Tom Shakespeare, is to put in place measures so that the practice of PGD, as it is practiced in a particular society, is not discriminatory towards disabled people.

John Harris argues that the expressivist objection is logically flawed, as choosing not to bring disabled people into the world does not logically imply devaluing existing people. (Harris 2005) On the basis of this consideration Harris simply dismisses the objection. Holm, though, correctly pointed out how considerations of logical necessity such as the one raised by Harris are largely irrelevant outside academia. (Holm 2008) Moreover, while it is possible to conceive in theory of a "socially embedded practice of prenatal diagnosis and termination of pregnancy that did not, as an empirical fact about that practice, express any negative attitudes towards the disabled and could not justifiably be construed to express such negative attitudes" (Holm 2008, 25) (as for example in a particular context, where the problem of allocation of scarce resources did not exist), this scenario is not the one, or not even close, to the one we have at the moment in our society. Instead, it is plausible to say that at least to some degree, our current practices of prenatal diagnosis and termination of pregnancy do express those attitudes that disability scholars claim. The burden of proof, therefore, rests on those who claim that current practices are not devaluing individuals with disabilities, not on individuals with disabilities to demonstrate that the practices are not devaluing them. Indeed, Holm notes that it is justified for individuals with disabilities to draw certain inferences (about the devaluing of themselves) from practices aimed at not conceiving individuals with such disabilities, as such inferences seem to be epistemically warranted (Holm 2008, 25). As an example, Holm offers the image of burning a flag: people seeing a flag being burnt are justified in drawing the inference about the symbolic meaning attached to the action, unless explicitly stated otherwise (for example, it would need to be clear that those burning a flag were doing it within the context of a "flag burning" festival, where flags of all nationalities where being burnt, or something like that where the traditional symbolic meaning attached to burning a flag would be displaced by another, new meaning). Not only do I find myself intuitively agreeing with Holm on this point, but I would also add that explaining away the devaluing of individuals with disabilities with logical necessity would probably not be sufficient, as Harris offers, but practical changes would be asked for. I will take a closer look at the expressivist arguments when I discuss DeGrazia (2012) in section 2.5.

Value pluralism

The second objection ("value pluralism") is a very powerful objection to classical eugenics practices, which subordinated the "good" of the individual to the "good" of the state that was considered objective and univocal. In this sense, contemporary eligogenic practices seem to be distant from classical ones, as parents are able to choose subjective conceptions of the good (e.g. deafness, achondroplasia), at least in countries where the approach to PGD is more permissive. Of course, the possibility of societal pressures or of cultural complicity, as pointed out by Little, is not to be dismissed. (Little 1998) See also the discussion of the following objection.

Coercion

As to the problem of coercion, it would seem easy to dismiss this concern at first sight as invalid in contemporary practices of reproductive genetic choices. The parents claim that they exercise their autonomy, right to self-determination and reproductive freedom in deciding whether to undergo IVF or PGD. Current eligogenics practices are not socially enforced, contrary to the positive and negative measures implemented in classical eugenics. As defined by Beauchamp and Childress, "coercion occurs if and only if one person intentionally used a credible and severe threat of harm or force to control another." (Beauchamp and Childress 2001) Along these lines, a subjective response in which individuals comply with a practice because they feel threatened does not qualify as coercion. I agree which Beauchamp and Childress, who criticize the tendency in contemporary biomedical ethics debate to render "coercion" an all-purpose term of ethical criticism. Other terms that should be used are persuasion, where a person is led to believe in something through the merit of reasons, and manipulation, where persons are swayed into doing what the manipulator wants by means other than coercion or persuasion, e.g. informational manipulation. (Beauchamp and Childress 2001) It needs to be noted that some kinds of current social "pressure" toward the best possible children could be described as forms of persuasion or manipulation. To what extent does the society in which these practices occur persuade or manipulate parents into taking such measures – to screen for children who have traits that mirror the values of that particular society? Robert Sparrow (2011) points out the pervasiveness of this problem in the practices of contemporary eugenics (see discussion below), and Margaret Olivia Little already mentioned above was the first scholar to identify the perils of cultural complicity inherent in enhancement technologies. (Little 1998)

Statism

The objection of "Statism" refers to the role of the State in shaping individuals' wishes and desires. Some distinctions though need to be drawn concerning the validity of this objection to contemporary eligogenic practices. As Suter pointed out, while a distinction is often drawn between eugenics and what she refers to as "neougenics" insofar as the former had the interests of the State as its goal, while the latter has the interests of the individuals (Suter 2007, 946), such an analysis is over-simplifying, as a closer look reveals that in both periods, the motives were actually mixed. Writes Suter:

> The classic rationale for eugenic sterilization included benefits to the sterilized individual … Just as classic eugenics was not motivated solely by social well-being, current and future reproductive technologies are advocated not solely to allow individuals to make decisions compatible with their values and goals. The technologies are also promoted and encouraged as socially responsible. (Suter 2007, 946)

Similar arguments supporting contemporary eligogenics practices and based on the promotion of a common societal good can also be found in the consequentialist arguments that some genetic enhancements will increase the total welfare of society, by increasing the percent of fit people in society. This kind of argument leads to the discussion of differential access to the enhancement technologies, and to the last objection identified by Buchanan and co-authors, i.e. the problem of justice or equality.

Justice

The fifth and last issue identified by Buchanan and co-authors, "justice," hinges on two problems: a) the problem of distribution of burdens and benefits in the eugenics programs, where the most disadvantaged were always the target of the eugenic policies which made them even worse off; and b) to the problem of equality of access to the technologies. As pointed out by Sparrow:

> The real danger posed by the development of effective technologies of human enhancement is not that religious conservatives will prevent couples from making use of these technologies, but that parents will eventually have no choice but to make use of them. Without them, their children will stand no chance of competing effectively in the world. (Sparrow 2011, 40)

The analysis by Sparrow is important as it points to a very concrete consequence of the use of genetic technologies to choose what kind of children to bring into the world. Even if there is no coercion from the State and parents are free to exercise their choices (to the point that they are free to choose traits traditionally considered "disabilities"), the pressures exercised by society and the problem of cultural complicity need to be taken into account when evaluating the ethical permissibility of genetic technologies for selective reproduction. Sparrow points out also the "very unattractive consequences" that we would have to accept if we endorsed some of the libertarian claims made by Harris and Savulescu, who argue in favour of a moral obligation, or duty, to bring into the world the best possible people. (Savulescu 2005; Savulescu 2007; Harris 2007; Harris 2012). One of these "very unattractive consequences" would be the increase in cultural complicity with socially problematic practices of discrimination towards minorities and conformism towards a "dominant" conception of the good. Quoting again Sparrow:

> In many parts of the world today, prevailing social circumstances are likely to have a much greater impact on the welfare of individuals than are other environmental factors. When thinking about which genes are best for our children, then, Harris and Savulescu's argument implies that we should take these factors into account. Thus, for instance, in a racist society, where children born with particular racial markers – skin color, hair type, shape of nose and lips, presence or absence of an epicanthic fold, and so on – will have reduced life prospects, a proper concern for their children's well-being requires that parents work to mitigate the impact of racism by altering the child's environment, or by manipulating the genes associated with these markers, or both. … Unfortunately, it will often be much easier to alter a child's genetics than the social conditions that will shape the ultimate impact of their genetics. (Sparrow 2011, 35)

Are we ready to accept this "repugnant conclusion" (borrowing from (Parfit 1984)) as a consequence of our obligation to enhance? As pointed out again by Sparrow, in many parts of Europe, North America, and Australia, this would probably mean that prospective parents would use PGD to bring into the world "white male children who would grow up to be tall and (probably) blonde haired and blue eyed." (Sparrow 2011, 35) Recently the Silicon Valley company 23&Me made the headlines after patenting a computerized process for selecting gamete donors to achieve a child with a "phenotype of interest" with in vitro fertilization.[5] Sparrow would presumably be concerned at how prospective parents could use this computerized process, although the company has denied all claims that it would be used to "design babies" for eugenics purposes. (Grant 2013)

Nicholas Agar indirectly replied to Sparrow and his concern over contemporary eugenics practices in his book "Liberal Eugenics. In defense of human enhancement." (Agar 2008, 5) Agar argues that the main difference between liberal eugenics and what he refers to as "authoritarian eugenics" is that the former is grounded in the principle of liberal societies (for which there are many and often incompatible ideas of the good life and of human flourishing), while the latter says that individuals should be left free to pursue their own idea with the tool of enhancement technologies. Agar's conception of liberal eugenics is not, though, to be unbounded or unregulated. On the contrary: while individuals should be left free to pursue and choose with whom to mate/to reproduce, they should not be left completely free to choose what kind of children to have. This is because, according to Agar, in the latter endeavour individuals will need to resort to the assistance of the state (or of a private organization) which can and should impose conditions in this cooperation, "refusing to assist reproductive choices that are morally defective in some significant ways" (Agar 2008, 16). As examples of these morally defective choices, Agar includes the "very unattractive consequences" pointed out by Sparrow, as choosing to have a straight child instead of a possibly gay one, or choosing to have a white child instead of a black one. Doing so would contribute to reinforcing ethically problematic societal practices, such as racism. Therefore, from a liberal viewpoint such as Agar's, the new freedom of choice opened up by new genetic technologies can be seen as an extension of parental reproductive freedom, which could be bounded in "morally defective cases." The judgment on the "moral defectiveness" needs to be made on a case-by-case analysis, though not further explored by Agar in his book.

---

5   http://blog.23andme.com/news/a-23andme-patent/ [accessed July 18, 2014]

Suter is also in favour of a contemporary eligogenic practice:

> Some of the attitudes and concerns of eugenics remain today - a focus on
> the heritability of traits, a tendency toward genetic determinism, a privileg-
> ing of science, a focus on societal benefits of genetic technologies, and most
> important, societal pressure to increase the chances of having "well-born"
> children or to decrease the incidence of "less fit" children. ... I argue that
> the propriety of neoeugenics, or eugenics for that matter, depends on moti-
> vation, context, and results; it cannot easily be categorized as always or never
> problematic. (Suter 2007, 948)

I agree with Suter's point on the necessity of a contextual analysis of
contemporary eligogenic practices to spell out all the dimensions of the use
of a particular genetic technology by parents to select specific traits. Indeed,
this is what I try to do in analysing genetic technologies used to choose what
kind of children to bring into the world (sections 2.4 and 2.5 in this chapter),
and in my analysis of the use of genetic technologies to scout out children's
talent. (sections 3.3 and 3.4) Finally, other important objections to eligogenics
practices aimed at "choosing children" can be raised in terms of what values we
are leaving to future generations. The possibility of exacerbating inequalities,
and of differential access between people who can avail themselves of genetic
technologies and others who cannot, are also pressing questions. Moreover,
as already noted above in the case of PGD, the discrepancies in regulation
of genetic technologies among countries provide the conditions for medical
and reproductive tourism within and outside Europe, further exacerbating the
problem of equality of access. (Meghani 2011; Zanini 2011)

To conclude this section, it seems to me that current eligogenic practices
are indeed morally problematic, but on different grounds than the possible
consequences on the future of our species. They seem to me to be problematic as they may infringe on children's right to an open future, on their developing autonomy, and on their possibilities of human flourishing (of "*eudamo-
nia*"). In addition, they seem to be problematic as they participate in the issue
of cultural complicity described above. In the next section I will a closer look
at the conflict that may arise in the context of genetic technologies between
parental procreative liberty and children's interest.

2.3 Procreative liberty, and self-determination

Individuals resort to genetic technologies to engage in new ways to reproduce. They also avail themselves of genetic technologies to shape the creation of what kind of people to bring into existence. Both these actions can be considered within the scope of "reprogenetics" borrowing from Silver who coined the term in his 1997 book "Remaking Eden." (Silver 1997) These kinds of choices take place both at the pre-natal and at the post-natal level. In this section and the following one I will focus on the former, while in sections 3.1 and 3.2 I will consider the latter.

"Procreative liberty" (PL) has been defined by Robertson as a "liberty or claim-right to decide whether or not to reproduce."[6] (Robertson 2003, 447) Robertson distinguishes between two components of PL: a negative component, and a positive component. The negative component amounts to the liberty to avoid reproducing, which includes the liberty to "avoiding intercourse, using contraceptives, refusing the transfer of embryos to the uterus, discarding embryos, terminating pregnancies, and being sterilized" (Roberston 2003, 447) The positive component amounts to the liberty to reproduce which involves "the freedom to take steps or make choices that result in the birth of biologic offspring, such as having intercourse, providing gametes for artificial or in vitro conception, placing embryos in the uterus, preserving gametes or embryos for later use, and avoiding the use of contraception, abortion, or sterilization." (Roberston 2003, 447) Each component has an independent justification and can be conceived as a different claim-right. Like most rights in a liberal society, the PL claim-right is to be understood primarily as a negative right, i.e., a right against interference by the state or others with reproductive decisions. A positive right of PL would entail a heavier burden on the state, i.e., to provide resources for assisted reproduction, facilities, infertility treatment, abortion, etc. While PL has both negative and positive components, in what follows I will concentrate on when we should refrain from interfering with PL, therefore on the negative component.

Why is PL so important? Buchanan and co-authors identify the interests

---

6   In this work I use the terms "reproductive freedom" and "procreative liberty" as synonyms.

and values that determine the moral importance of PL, namely self-determination, individual good or wellbeing (the precise form of this argument depending on the account of wellbeing chosen), and equalitiy of expectation and opportunity. (Buchanan et al. 2000, 204–256) Self-determination is defined as the interest of an individual in making significant decisions about one's own life, according to own values or conceptions of a good life. It is also important to note, as pointed out by Robertson (2003), that recognizing the importance of PL (or even recognizing it as a moral or legal right) does not mean that it is an absolute value that cannot ever be overriden. Rather, it means that there is "a *strong presumption* [emphasis, added] in its favor, with the burden on opponents to show that there is a good case for limiting it." (Robertson 2003, 448) If this is the case, when is it justified to drop the presumption, and interfere with PL? Before answering this question I first distinguish between six aspects of the scope of PL, following the analysis by Buchanan et al., (2000):

> The choice of whether to procreate, with whom, and by what means;
> The choice of when to procreate;
> The choice of how many children to have;
> The choice of what kind of children to have;
> The choice of whether to have biologically related children;
> The social conditions that support reproductive choices.
> (Buchanan et al. 2000, 204–256)

Buchanan and co-authors note how a justified interference may be specific only to one component or another of PL. Genetic technologies used for current eligogenic practices focus on the fourth component of PL, i.e. the choice of what kind of children to bring into the world. This, though, seems to be a component more closely related to the determinations of others, than to one's self-determination, and the overall moral case for determining what another is like is substantially weaker than the moral case for determining how one's life should be. I apply this argument to object to the use of pre-implantation genetic diagnosis to choose what kind of children to bring into the world, in a paper where I analyse the case of parents that use PGD to choose a trait traditionally considered a disability: deafness, (Camporesi 2010) and included in this work in a slightly revised form in the next section.

2.4 Choosing deafness with preimplantation genetic diagnosis: an ethical way to carry on a cultural bloodline?[7]

> Consider the theoretical possibility of screening to ensure that only a disabled child would be conceived. This would surely be monstrous. And we think it would be monstrous because we do not believe it is just as good to be born with a disability.

These words were written by ethicist Jonathan Glover in his paper "Future People, Disability and Screening" in 1992. (Glover 1992) Whereas screening and choosing for a disability remained a theoretical possibility twenty or so years ago, it has now become reality. In 2008, Susannah Baruch and colleagues at John Hopkins University published a survey of 190 American PGD clinics, and found that 3% reported having the intentional use of PGD "to select an embryo for the presence of a disability."(Baruch, Kaufman, and Hudson 2008) Even before, in 2002, a controversy was generated by the case of Candace A. McCullough and Sharon M. Duchesneau, a lesbian and deaf couple from Maryland who set out to have a deaf child by intentionally soliciting a deaf sperm donor. (Spriggs 2002)

The discourse on using PGD in order to choose what kind of children to bring into the world has been monopolized by the discussion of the different notions of "disability" and by the related topic of the treatment–enhancement distinction. In this discourse, different definitions of "disability" seem to imply different normative judgments about parental reproductive choices. I choose here to adopt a different perspective, and to shift the debate from the level of disability to that of "impairment." I will argue that it is still possible to claim that choosing deafness with PGD is morally wrong, without arguing that deafness is a disability, but framing the case in terms of justice toward the future children and limitation of a reasonably broad array of different life plans. I also support my view in terms of the balance between self-

---

7   This section first appeared with the same title in a slightly modified form in *Cambridge Quarterly of Healthcare Ethics* (2010), 19, 86–96. doi:10.1017/S0963180109990272

determination of parents within their sphere of reproductive freedom and their determination of future children.

Different Regulations

Deafness is the most common sensory disorder, present in one of every 500 newborns. (Hilgert, Smith, and Van Camp 2009) With almost fifty genes implicated in nonsyndromic hearing loss, it is also an extremely heterogeneous trait. The most frequent genes implicated in autosomal recessive nonsyndromic hearing loss are GJB2, the gene for connexin 26 (Cx26), followed by SLC26A4, MYO15A, OTOF, CDH23, and TMC1. A Cx26 mutation can be detected in ~30% of sporadic cases of prelingual hearing impairment. The likelihood of detection of a Cx26 mutation increases to more than half of the families with identified autosomal recessive transmission. Up to 95% of deaf children are born to parents with normal hearing. (Hilgert, Smith, and Van Camp 2009)

Countries have adopted very different legal approaches to the regulation of PGD. The United States has no federal regulation at all, but PGD issues are regulated by professional standards. In Canada, sex selection is permitted only to prevent the transmission of a genetic disease. (Deonandan and Bente 2014).[8] In Australia, PGD is regulated partly by state legislation and partly under the National Health and Medical Research Council guidelines on the use of assisted reproductive technology (NHMRC ART Guidelines). Europe is very heterogenous in this respect, as laws range from prohibitive (PGD is not allowed in Austria, Ireland, and Italy, and only in very limited cases in Germany since July 2011) to restrictive (where PGD is permitted only in cases of screening for disorders or in cases of tissue typing, as in Scandinavian countries, Spain, Belgium, and France). The lack of harmonized regulation at the European level has resulted in an increasing number of couples crossing borders seeking PGD. (Soini 2007; Zanini 2011) The UK approach is certainly the most liberal, as PGD is allowed also for tissue typing and for screening for disease susceptibilities. In the UK, PGD is licensed by the Human Embryology and Fertilization Authority (HFEA) for around fifty conditions, including cystic fibrosis, familial hypercholesterolemia, blood disorders such as thalas-

---

8   At the time of writing, July 2014.

semia and hemophilia, muscular dystrophy, deafness, achondroplasia, Down syndrome, Huntington's Chorea, X-linked mental retardation and other X-linked disorders, and so forth.[9] (HFEA 2013) For an up-to-date comparative review of assisted reproduction and PGD policies, see (Deonandan and Bente 2014).

In spring 2008, the debate on choosing children with a "disability" surfaced again in the UK on Clause 14(4) (9) of the draft of Human Fertilization and Embryology Bill, which stated that "embryos" known to have a genetic abnormality "with a significant risk of transmitting a serious mental or physical disability, serious illness, or any other serious medical condition … must not be preferred to those that are not known to have such an abnormality." (Wales Online 2008) A petition was filed to drop the clause 14(4) (9) of the HFE bill, and was rejected on August 20, 2008, on the ground that "[i]t is in the best interests of the child not to prefer embryos that have a significant risk of developing a serious medical condition." ("Petition Against Clause 14(4) (9) of HFE Bill and Government Response" 2008) The consequent debate revolved around the interpretation of the clause and its relevance for the deafness case, because, according to one interpretation, it could imply that a deaf couple undergoing PGD would not be able to choose embryos carrying a gene associated with a genetic hearing impairment.

The Impairment–Disability Distinction

Do we need to define "deafness" as a disability to argue that it is morally wrong to choose deaf children with PGD? And do different definitions imply different normative judgments about the ethical acceptability of parental choices regarding genetic traits? In that follows I will try to provide an answer to the first question and make some suggestions relevant to the second one.

There are several notions of disability: a purely medical definition such as the one given by the World Health Organization (WHO), (World Health

---

9   The list of conditions for which PGD is allowed is constantly revised and updated, and more conditions are awaiting consideration at the time of writing. See [http://www.hfea.gov.uk/cps/hfea/gen/pgd-screening.htm] [accessed July 18, 2014]

Organization 2001) a purely social definition such as the one formulated by Michael Oliver (Oliver 1996) and a "harmed-condition" account of disability by John Harris. (Harris 2007, 91-93) Here I do not wish to argue in favor of a particular notion of disability, but I take as a premise a particular notion and then shift the discussion to the level of impairment. As Jonathan Glover also argued in his book *Choosing Children. Genes, Disability and Design*, it is time to abandon the "unfruitful" disability debate. (Glover 2007) On the one hand, "disability" is defined as the possible functional consequence of impairment (e.g., inability to hear certain sounds or inability to speak clearly). (World Health Organization 2001) This definition is close to the commonsense notion of disability and impairment. On the other hand, the 2001 revision of the WHO's International Classification of Functioning, Disability and Health defines "impairment" as "an abnormality of a structure or function of the body" that can be congenital (present at birth) or acquired, through disease or trauma. According to the definition by Oliver, impairment is "lacking part or all of a limb, or having a defective limb, organ or mechanism of the body," whereas "disability" is defined as "the disadvantage or restriction of activity caused by a contemporary social organization which takes no or little account of people who have physical impairments and thus excludes them from participation in the mainstream of social activities."(Oliver 1996, 22) Therefore, accepting Oliver's view, impairment has to do exclusively with the body; while disability also necessarily involves other factors. While impairments often result in disabilities, they need not necessarily do so. A disability is inherently relational: being disabled is being unable to do something, to perform some significant range of tasks or functions that individuals in some reference groups (e.g., adults) are ordinarily able to do. How do these notions of disability, and of impairment relate to the deafness case? Being deaf in a deaf community is not a disability understood in these terms, but is still an impairment. In other words, one can have a physical impairment without being disabled, for example, a person in a wheelchair living in a town devoid of architectonic barriers. For this reason someone's race, ethnicity or sexual preference is not a disability under a social constructivist approach, precisely because all its disadvantages are socially imposed, but can become so in particular societies.

Deafness as a "variation"?

Empirical research suggests that deaf people often have a degree of preference for a deaf child, and a rather smaller number would consider acting on
their preference with the use of selective techniques. (Middleton, Hewison,
and Mueller 1998; Stern et al. 2002) It turns out that such parents do not view
certain genetic conditions as disabilities, but as a passport to enter into a rich,
shared culture. They see being deaf as defining their cultural identity and sign
language as a sophisticated, unique form of communication. Parents contend
that not hearing is just a form of human variation, and one that has given rise
to a culture of its own, with members who want to see their community continuing into the future. (Mundy 2002)

Darshak M. Sanghavi, a pediatric cardiologist at the University of
Massachusetts Medical School, supports the parental choices:

> Controlling a child's genetic makeup, even to preserve what some would
> consider a disease, is the latest tactic of parents in an increasingly globalized
> society where identity seems besieged and in need of aggressive preservation.
> Traditionally, cultures were perpetuated through assortative mating, with
> intermarriage among the like-minded and the like appearing. … Viewed in
> this context, the use of PGD to select for deafness may be merely *another
> ritual to ensure that one's children carry on a cultural bloodline.* (emphasis added)
> (Sanghavi 2006)

According to many deaf parents, deafness is a condition that opens up as
many and as valuable options as it closes down. In this sense, they argue,
deafness is analogous to an ethnic minority status, as both communities suffer
socially imposed disadvantages because of their condition, in particular social
contexts. But is it plausible to claim that not hearing is equivalent to an ethnic
minority status? I contend that it is not, on the ground that deafness is an
impairment that limits a broad array of different life plans, independently of
the social context.

Let us, then, imagine how Oliver's definitions could be applied if we lived
in a much more liberal and nondiscriminatory society than ours. Of course,
it is true that different shades of disability could go with certain impairment,

depending on the social context, but the hearing impairment would still be limiting the person in some activities even in the most advanced societies, whereas the social constraints imposed on other kinds of minorities would disappear because they are completely socially determined. Thus, under Oliver's account, being deaf would still be an impairment in any kind of society, because of the underlying asymmetry of this trait. Therefore, even accepting a social constructivist model of disability and defining deafness as an impairment which does not necessarily go with a disability, the question whether it is morally wrong to choose children with a physical impairment stays with us. Let us elaborate a bit more on this and imagine two groups of people living in an ideal society with no societal barriers toward deaf people. In this society, the only differences between the two groups would be that one group is able to hear and the other cannot; that one communicates with sign language and the other with a verbal, spoken language. Even in our progressive and nondiscriminatory society the relationship between the two groups would remain asymmetrical, as hearing people could be part of the deaf culture by learning how to communicate with sign language, but not vice versa. (Levy 2002) Of course, to this it can be objected that being born genetically deaf is not the same thing as learning to be deaf and learning the sign language. As Mackenzie and Scully have argued, the embodiment of a disability is the necessary premise to make certain ethical claims. (Mackenzie and Scully 2007) While I agree on this point, and on the point that the deaf culture may have its compensations that hearing people cannot fully experience, I still think that the fundamental point here is that deaf parents do not need to choose to exclude their children from the hearing world in order to include them in theirs (however imperfectly, as parents may counterargue), because both worlds and languages are open to their children: both the hearing and the not hearing worlds, both the verbal and the nonverbal languages. Tom Shakespeare made a very similar point in his most recent work: "There seem to be internal contradiction in the Deaf approach to cochlear implants. First, if Deafness has really nothing to do with impairment, then logically there would be no reason for Deaf people to oppose impairment reduction. Second, if Deafness is about being a member of a sign language community, there is nothing to stop hearing children of Deaf adults being members of that community too: indeed, there is a thriving Children of Deaf Adults (CODA) movement which enjoys membership in both Deaf and hearing world." (Shakespeare 2013, 152) Sanghavi also wrote that:

> The small number of PGD centers selecting for mutations doesn't bother me greatly. After all, even natural reproduction is an error-prone process … I've learned to respect a family's judgment. Many parents share a touching faith that having children similar to them will strengthen family and social bonds … . But it's not for me to say. (Sanghavi 2006)

While granting that parents have good intentions concerning the future of their children, I would like to question the equivalence between natural reproduction being an "error-prone process," and deliberately choosing to have a deaf child with PGD. In addition, even though I agree with Sanghavi that it should not be up to him or to individual practitioners to decide on these matters, it does not follow that it is up to nobody to decide. In other words, I think that there is still ground to argue that parental reproductive freedom should be regulated in some way, avoiding the technological Catch-22 mentioned before.

Why it is Morally Wrong to Choose Deafness with PGD

Framing the issue in terms of justice toward the future children avoids not only the thorny discussion of what a disability is but also the related and somewhat underlying discussion of the treatment – enhancement distinction. This distinction has been strongly criticized (for one, see Bortolotti and Harris 2006) and forces us to treat relevantly similar cases in dissimilar ways, by making some "morally arbitrary" *ad hoc* assumptions, as illustrated in 1.2. Such a distinction cannot play a moral role, because it is useless in helping us to draw both an obligatory/nonobligatory boundary and a permissible/impermissible boundary.

In our society, there is a presumption in favor of not interfering with parents' decisions, and they are allowed a large degree of discretion in choosing what is good for their children (e.g., education, religion). (Buchanan et al. 2000, 156–8) Some argue that this should not be the case (and parents should be licensed by the state, as it is required from people applying for an adoption). (LaFollette 2010) Other scholars have made the case for compulsory parental education, a less extreme proposal to which I am sympathetic. (Bortolotti and Cutas 2009)

Reproductive freedom is one of the fundamental rights of the person and finds its justification (at least in part) in the democratic presumption. (Buchanan et al. 2000, 204–222; Harris 2007, 72–4) According to this principle, citizens should be free to live according to their own values, and the state should not interfere with their freedom unless there is a direct danger to other citizens or to society in general. Note that it is not sufficient that other people disagree with the choices of a person or find her values "fastidious" or "disgusting" for a limitation to freedom; otherwise all our fundamental freedoms of speech, expression, religion, sex, and reproduction would vanish together with the very concept of democracy.

This said, I believe that in case of parents choosing deaf children with PGD, the condition of a "direct danger to other citizens" (i.e., future children) is satisfied, and the state (through some authority such as HFEA in the United Kingdom) could, and indeed should, interfere with the parental reproductive freedom. The direct danger to the children would be the restriction of a broad array of possible, future life plans due to deafness. The extensive character of the hindrance makes the case for the limitation of the democratic presumption and therefore of the reproductive freedom, whereas it does not make the case for limiting parental freedom in more general terms (as other arguments would be needed to support such a claim). Along lines of reasoning similar to those by Buchanan and coauthors, I believe that a certain degree of neutrality must be expected from parents toward different conceptions of the good for their children. (Buchanan et al. 2000, 167–70) Parents, *qua persons*, can, of course, have a particular conception of the good and lead their lives according to it (which brings us back to the democratic presumption), but parents, *qua parents*, should maintain a certain degree of neutrality toward different conceptions of the good for their children. In other words, parents should not be allowed to make their children suitable for only one particular conception of a good life that the parents happen to have, such as the conception of the rich and shared culture of the deaf community. Any intervention that would greatly restrict this range of choices, as a hearing impairment would do, would be unjust to the child.

Finally, the notion of "self-determination" is one of the values that determines the moral importance of reproductive freedom (together with individual wellbeing, equality of expectations, and opportunities. (Buchanan et al. 2000, 204–22) Self-determination can be understood as the interest in making significant decisions about one's own life for oneself, according to one's own values and conception of a good life. John Rawls characterized this interest as based on people's capacity to form, revise over time, and pursue a plan of life and conception of the good. (Rawls 1971) This said, the impact of peoples' actions on others (i.e., future children) must be understood as a competing moral consideration that can, and must, place a limit on the parents' self determination and, therefore, on their reproductive freedom. Shaping the nature of children is not primarily a matter of individual self-determination but as well, and more importantly, the determination of another. I would like to stress here that I am not questioning the motivations of the parents reported and interpreted by Sanghavi. Such parents may all have good intentions – and thinking to choose "the best" for their children – when choosing to have a deaf child through PCD, but considerations of justice suggest that parents should not maintain their currently accorded discretion toward such broad scope capabilities such as hearing, because this would factually amount to determine the lives of others.

I am aware that an important problem of threshold is looming in the background here, namely: Where should the threshold be set, and when could reproductive freedom be limited, on the basis of justice considerations and the limitation of a reasonable array of different life plans? In section 3.4 I discuss the case of parents using genetic technologies (direct-to-consumer genetic tests) to supposedly measure their children's talents, and steering their education aggressively in the direction of pre-professionalisation of sport on the basis of the results of these tests.

The Social Construction of Impairment

So far, my arguments have been based on the definition of disability and impairment by Michael Oliver. One objection could be raised on the basis of the more radical claim that impairment is also socially constructed. Cole (2007) argues that disability arises always in a particular social context and that the combination of "social structure + impairment" causes the disability.

Certainly, the disability is the product of the interaction between bodily impairment and social context, but it is the social context that gives the action
or ability its form and context. (Cole 2007, 172)

Cole concludes that "it is the political idea of disability that determines what
counts as bodily impairment," (Cole 2007, 175) because persons wearing
glasses to correct some minor eyesight defect have an "eyesight that is impaired to some extent" (at least he concedes this point!) but we "would not
want to describe them as bodily impaired." (Cole 2007, 175)

I would like to remark on two points touched upon by Cole that are useful
for the discussion of the deafness case. The first revolves around the issue of
the normativity of definitions. Cole aims at defining "deafness" or "blindness"
as "something less than an impairment," as a "mere inability," with the purpose
of deriving a normative judgment about the permissibility of making some
kinds of parental choices or of society adopting certain kinds of policies. But
the derivation of ethical prescriptions from a definition cannot be taken as
straightforward, it requires a justification. Therefore, while we could accept
Cole's point that under some circumstances deafness would not count as an
impairment, no ethical judgment about PGD screening permissibility could
be automatically derived. Secondly, I do not think it is necessary to define
"deafness" as disability, impairment or inability to infer some kind of ethical
judgment on the parental choices. In other words, it is not necessary to possess
a normative definition to argue that choosing deafness with PGD is morally
wrong. Indeed, it can still be argued that it is wrong to choose deafness with
PGD even if it is not defined as an impairment on the ground that there is
an underlying asymmetry between hearing and non hearing people, and that
not hearing is a broad limitation of the future child's life plans. Even disability
rights scholar Tom Shakespeare writes along similar lines objecting to a radical
social model of disability: "… Even in the most accessible world practical,
there will always be residual disadvantage attached to many impairments"
(Shakespeare 2013, 42) and in addition, with specific reference to the case of
deaf parents choosing to have deaf children as quoted above, he has written
along similar lines as mine of the existence of an intrinsic asymmetry between
hearing and non hearing people. (Shakespeare 2013, 152)

To conclude: as defined by Oliver, deafness remains an impairment, even if in some societies, and in deaf communities, it may not count as a disability. Parents who choose to impose on their children their idiosyncratic vision of the good, be it in relation to the deaf culture or to some other conceptions of the good, are acting unjustly toward the future child, who should have a sufficiently large array of opportunities to decide on her own what is good for her later in life. Moreover, the advantages of being part of a deaf community are asymmetric, as also a hearing person could learn the sign language and be part of it (even if only "imperfectly"). To those scholars, like Phillip Cole, who view "impairment" as socially constructed, I replied that we could abandon the quest for a normative definition valid for several traits (e.g., deafness, dwarfism, blindness) and reason on a case by case basis. In other words, we can decide to call deafness simply "deafness": Is it or is it not "not being able to hear"? If we agree on this, then we should agree that it is a limitation on the future of the child, and not a minor one, as it is a broad capability and a necessary condition for a vast array of plans of life. In other words, I am adopting here a critical realist perspective as the one adopted by Tom Shakespeare (2013), where he recognizes medicine will never completely erase the problems and limitation of embodiment, and that impairment is a condition that sooner or later faces each one of us faces in life (in this sense, we are all "temporarily abled").

What are the consequences of my claim? Should parental reproductive freedom in terms of PGD choices be regulated from a legal point of view? What about parental discretion for other kinds of choices? Where should we put the threshold, if we decide that we need one (as I argued)? And who decides?

I cannot here respond fairly to these complex questions and will only suggest two possible directions to elaborate elsewhere. For what concerns regulation, the issue here is subtle and manifold: As Sanghavi (2006) rightly noticed, humans have always been mating the "alike" to have children like them. I believe this kind of reproductive freedom should not be constrained, as we would not want to live in a paternalistic society where deaf couples are discouraged from having children for the "good" of future generation or for improving the gene pool, as was done with forced sterilization back in the classical eugenics period. Somehow different is the case of the lesbian couple who seeked a deaf donor to have a very high probability (although not a certainty, because of the heterogeneity of the genetic trait) to conceive a deaf child, as Candace and Sharon McCullough did. Can this still be considered a kind of assortative mating? I doubt it.

The case is even more straightforward for parents who choose PGD to be "sure" (medical errors not considered) to have a deaf child. Unlike Sanghavi, I do think that there is a morally relevant difference between the natural errors of reproduction and the intentional choice to have a deaf child. This morally relevant difference makes the case for the justified natural assortative mating, but it does not make it for cases of PGD screening for deafness or of couples soliciting a deaf donor. Finally, who would be entitled to limit parental reproductive freedom, and on which authority? Such a decision should not rest on the shoulders (and discretion!) of individual practitioners, as Sanghavi pointed out. Exactly for this reason the UK and other countries have developed institutions to regulate such issues, such as Human Fertilization and Embryology in the United Kingdom.

I am willing to accept the consequences of a consistent application of this line of thought, including further limitations on parental discretion concerning other kinds of interventions that could limit a reasonable array of different life plans of the future children. Decisions in terms of education (e.g., is it justified for parents belonging to the Amish community to withdraw their children from school at 14 years, two years before the normal age limit for compulsory education? (Mameli 2007)), religion (e.g., should parents be allowed to impose their choice of religion of their children) could also fall within those that need to be regulated.

2.5 Disabilities, or just differences? An analysis of the expressivist objection

In the last section of this chapter I consider an alternative way of framing the case of choosing deafness with PGD based on the "expressivist objection" that deafness is only a "difference," and not a disability. According to the expressivist objection, traits such as dyslexia, deafness, achondroplasia are not to be considered disabilities, but mere differences. Such traits, the objection goes, are not more disadvantageous *per se* than being born black in the U.S. South in the 19th century, or being gay in contemporary Ughanda, as it is the social structure that confers on these traits their disadvantage. From this perspective, all disadvantages are contingent on the socio- and cultural context the individual finds herself in. Those who resort to this argument reject the medical model of disability (according to which disability is a relatively long-lasting, biologically grounded condition that impairs the individual in one or more significant ways) and adopt the social model of disability, which maintains that disability involves a loss or limitation of opportunities due to institutional or social barriers. As already mentioned above, Mackenzie and Scully argue that a particular embodiment is a necessary condition to make claims about one's own quality of life, and therefore that the incorporation of narratives of the disabled individuals becomes a necessary step when deliberating about PGD. They write:

> We do not dispute that the capacity for imaginative projection, or simulation, is central to our ability to understand other people's mental states. However, there is a significant gap between the kinds of simple cases of belief and desire attribution about which philosophers of mind are concerned, and imaginatively entering into another's point of view sufficient to understand, for example, how that person experiences disability or evaluates her quality of life. (Mackenzie and Scully 2007, 339–40)

Scully also points out the potential exacerbations of equality of existing problems of access to the genetic technologies, and of differential treatment in society that could be raised by the use of preimplantation genetic diagnosis to prevent individuals with disability to come into the world. (Scully 2008)

I am sympathetic with the writings of Tom Shakespeare, who is a disability rights scholar and a disabled person affected by achondroplasia and skeletal displasia. Along similar lines to what I argued in the previous section, Tom is not concerned with the diagnosis or the label given to a particular condition, but with the very real and concrete consequences arising from the condition. He writes:

> Diagnosis is not my problem, and nor is the label which you give to my skeletal dysplasia/restricted growth/dwarfism/achondroplasia, let alone my

spinal cord injury and consequent neuropathic pain. My problem is my physical embodiment and my experience of negative symptoms arising from my
impairment. ... I want to say that impairment and illness is often experienced
not just as a difference, but as difficulty and limitation and pain and suffering.
... *Having an impairment is not like being gay or from a different culture: the solution
is not just revaluing diversity.* (emphasis added) (Shakespeare 2013, 66-67, 84)

Therefore, as it is clear from the quote above, while the conditions of society
have of course a substantial impact on the lives of those with an impairment, even the elimination of all social barriers would not eliminate all the
symptoms inherent in a condition. This is what is known as a "critical realist
perspective." DeGrazia objects to the argument that disabilities are not only
"differences" with an excursion into value theory that takes into account the
voices of many people with major disabilities, who claim nonethless to be
happy with their lives. (DeGrazia 2012, 108) As a matter of fact, disabled
individuals often assert that the disability adds value to their lives, that it made
them "better persons," and that if they could choose to be born again without
the disabilities, they would not do so. What weight should this kind of claim
be given in relation to the discussion of cases such as that of individuals resorting to PGD to choose deafness?

Some authors object to these narratives by arguing that individuals with
major disabilities are subject to self-deception as an unconscious objection to
cope with their difficult lives. This, though, does not seem to be a successful
strategy for at least two reasons: a) it is quite a common phenomenon for
individuals with disabilities to argue that they are happy with their lives and b)
the presumption should be that the best judge of what is best for one's own
life is the individual living that life. I agree with the analysis by DeGrazia, who
is cautious in attributing self-deception to individuals. He writes: "Generally
speaking, it is the person herself who best knows how her life is going for her."
(DeGrazia 2012, 112) Even if DeGrazia acknowledges that some individuals
may think they are satisfied with their lives as a consequence of the dampening
of their desires due to the loss of functioning they experience, this judgment
of "comparative achievement might not be relevant to the issue of how well
the subject's life is going for her." (ibid) Therefore, on the one hand, DeGrazia
adopts subjectivist theories of values in contrast to objectivist theories of

values, which he argues are 'theoretically presumptuous" and require a heavy burden of justification. On the other hand, though, DeGrazia does not accept subjectivist accounts of value *tout court*. In order to avoid the seemingly absurd implication of subjectivism that a person is happy when all her beliefs are systematically and profoundly distorted (deluded individuals), we need to define happiness in a way that is more plausible than the mere reduction to either pleasurable feelings or desire-satisfaction. This more plausible definition is to define happiness in terms of "life-satisfaction," i.e., satisfaction with how one's life on the whole is going. Also, this would require a reality-based check, understood as: "a person's happiness makes her well-off only if it is based on a more or less accurate understanding of her circumstances." This reality check for DeGrazia avoids defining happy an individual who is subject to delusions.[10] To try to reconcile objectivist and subjectivist element of his account, DeGrazia argues that we should take into account the subjectivist report of individuals with disabilities and avoid the argument of self-deception. As an example (and a way out of disability discourses), DeGrazia introduces the case of the "happy slave": "If a slave is happy despite having no illusions about his situation then he has overcome the odds and is actually doing well. He is not less well-off just because his desires and expectations have been partly shaped by oppression." (DeGrazia 2012, 114) Other authors have discussed the apparent unsolvable contradiction of the happy slave case. Among these authors, Hannah Arendt's analysis seems to me to be able to capture better the nuances of the condition of happiness. Arendt distinguishes between two aspects of happiness of the slave: *eudaimonia*, defined as "an objective status depending first of all upon wealth and health" (something the slave could not enjoy by definition because they were subjected both to physical necessity and to man-made violence), and the actual subjective wellbeing as declared by the slave. (Arendt 1958, 31) The analysis by Arendt makes sense of the possibility that a slave – or another person in a severely disadvantage condition – could still claim to be "happy" without being deluded or subjected to self-deception, but could not possibility enjoy the possibility of human flourishing captured by the concept of eudaimonia.

---

10   I am not going to enter here into the discussion of delusions and happiness, to which I could not really contribute (see Bortolotti 2010).

Therefore, returning to the discussion of whether disability are just differences or not, we could say that disabilities need not be disadvantageous, as a person can fare just as well overall as a person without the disability, but it does not follow from this that disabilities are mere differences. "Disabilities involve the absence of a kind of functioning that plays a significant role in human life" (ibid, 115) and are *"presumptively disadvantageous"* [emphasis added] since they present an obstacle to wellbeing (even in the best possible societal scenario) but are not necessarily disadvantageous, for despite their obstacles, people can – and indeed, do – fare well. But if they do so, they have overcome their odds. To conclude, "because disabilities are presumptively disadvantageous, it must be considered harmful to inflict a disability on an individual" (115). In this sense, the arguments by DeGrazia are not too far from mine included in section 2.4, as I also argue that impairments such as deafness are disadvantageous for children. The right to an open future seems to be one of those arguments predominantly used in the context of children, while DeGrazia's analysis focuses more on arguments of individuals who reached adulthood with a disability.

We also need to acknowledge the increasingly prominent role and significance of patients' narratives in bioethics, which has been witnessing a shift in the last fifteen years from a "principled" default to a reflective mode, in particular in the analysis of the doctor/patient dilemma that arise at the bedside. (Lindemann 1997; Charon and Montello 2002) Though I will not enter here into this discussion, I would like to recognize the importance of incorporating, and giving proper weight, to the narratives of patients or individuals with disability when discussing the ethical permissibility of a particular technology such as for example PGD as used to choose to have deaf children "like themselves," quoting from Sanghavi (2006). This though does not mean that I would be prepared to accept the use of PGD to choose deafness, as I am of the opinion that the child's possibilities for a full human flourishing would be unjustly diminished. To reiterate, I am not saying here that the child could not grow up to be a happy and flourishing person, but if s/he did so, s/he would have done so at the expenses of an initial disadvantage.

In the next chapter I discuss genetic technologies applied to enhance athletic performance, discussing gene transfer, gene enhancement, and gene doping scenarios from a scientific, regulatory and ethical point of view. In the second part of the chapter I discuss the ethical and social implication of the recent boom of direct-to-consumer genetic tests to scout out children's athletic potential.

Chapter 3

From bench to track & field: Genetic technologies to enhance athletic performance

3.1 Gene transfer, gene enhancement and gene doping: infringing the spirit of sport?

Sport can be considered the first area where performance enhancement has been heavily regulated, and has thus served as one of the first testing grounds for enhancement technologies, for anti-enhancement regulation, and for public reaction to enhancement. Contrary to what may be thought, the administration of substances with the aim to enhance athletic performance has not always been viewed with a negative connotation, but is instead a relatively recent acquisition. For a long time, what we now consider "doping" was viewed as a legitimate way to extend the athlete's capabilities, and sport was seen as the experimental terrain *par excellence* where it was possible to do so. Trying to enhance one's own athletic performance with any available means was understood as the natural human reaction to coping with fatigue, and competition in sports was understood first as a challenge between athletes and fatigue, and only secondly between athletes and their competitors. The professional athlete was using her own body as the subject of experimentation, and the athlete herself became an experimental subject. This identification of the athlete's body with an experimental terrain can be dated back to 1894, when the pioneering French sports physician Philippe Tissié started administering several types of beverages to cyclists to test their value as performance enhancer. (Hoberman 2009) In this sense, Tissié was regarding the elite athlete as an experimental subject whose exertions and traumas could shed light onto the unexplained human physiology in a kind of reverse extrapolation from the track & field to the bedside. (Hoberman 2009)

This "functional view" of doping was promoted throughout the 1950s by a sharp distinction between amateur and professional athletes that does not exist anymore in our conception of sport. The professional athlete was seen as inhabiting a different moral universe in which the use of performance-enhancing drugs was tolerated, and promoted, because it was regarded as the only way for the individual professional athlete to win competitions, remain a professional athlete, and ultimately to make a living. This was not the case for the amateur athlete, who was considered the privileged one, and did not have to take on the risks associated with the consumption of often dangeours performance-enhancing substances. For this reason, the permission to dope was not accorded to the sports amateur, whose image became encapsulated as the British gentleman practising sports as a hobby, as a pastime. Going even further back in time, to the ancient Olympics, it is important to remember that the amount of time to be devoted to training before competition was severely constrained, on the basis of the same reasoning that the real athlete was not to be a professional, "menial" labourer, but a healthy person merely expressing natural talents. (Mathias 2004)

It is not easy to determine when and where the idea that doping violates the spirit of sport (the current stance of the World Anti-Doping Agency discussed below) came into existence. Plausibly, it was not something which emerged suddenly, but rather came into existence gradually in the first two decades of the 20th century. As noted by Hoberman, nationalism was one medium for the emergence of this idea, as in the first decade of the 20th century scientists were accusing each other across the Atlantic to hide the possession of a supposedly secret formula to combat fatigue. (Hoberman 2009) At the beginning of the 20th century, objections of "reprehensible doping" focused more on the medical dangers for the athlete's health than on the idea that doping was a form of cheating which would violate the spirit of sport. Then, in the 1920s and '30s, the idea that doping behaviours violated the ideals of sportsmanship as fair play emerged in parallel to the commercialization of sports and their increasing importance as mass culture. Though still in the 1950s, Sir Adolphe Abrahams, an Honorary Medical Officer to the International Athletics Board and the British Olympic Team, was expressing difficulties regarding how to distinguish between legitimate and less legitimate means to enhance athletic performance. He wrote:

It is not easy ... to draw the line where legitimate stimulation ends and reprehensible "doping" begins; the distinction is largely a matter of opinion and of conscience. (Abrahams 1958)

The Establishment of the World Anti-Doping Agency

The International Olympic Committee (IOC) established its first list of banned substances in 1967, and in 1999 convened the World Conference on Doping in Sport. This event, which can also be seen as a reaction to the widespread Tour de France doping scandals in 1998, led to the creation of the World Anti-Doping Agency (WADA), on November 10, 1999. WADA is based on the cooperation between sports organisations and governments, and is financed by sports organisations and governments on an equal basis.

In March 2003 WADA released its first World Anti-Doping Code (WADC), now in its 3rd revised edition. The rationale behind the WADC is to harmonise anti-doping rules and measures. Nearly all international sports federations have accepted the WADC, and governments support WADA financially. (McNamee and Tarasti 2010) WADA defines a substance as doping, and therefore prohibits it, if it meets two of the following three criteria:

It has the potential to enhance or enhances sports performance;
It represents an actual or potential risk to the athlete;
It violates the spirit of sport. (WADA Code 2012)

WADA is now in the process of revising its Code, expected to come into effect with a new version in 2015. I discuss the revisions and the desirability of a shift towards the inclusion of the necessary condition of performance enhancement in this work in section 3.5 and more at length in Camporesi and McNamee (2014).

In 2001, shortly after the creation of WADA, the IOC convened the first working group on gene doping. The group's finding affirmed support for the medical applications of gene therapy but advised taking measures to keep genetic modification out of the realm of sports. Quoting from the official WADA publication, "Play True":

We endorse the development and application of gene therapy for the prevention and treatment of human disease. However, we are aware that there is
the potential for abuse of gene therapy medicine and we shall begin to establish procedures and state-of-the-art testing methods for identifying athletes
who might misuse such technology. (Haisma and de Hon 2006)

In March 2002, the first workshop on gene doping was organized by WADA
at the Banbury Center in New York.[1] Shortly thereafter, in 2004, WADA also
created a "Gene Doping Expert Group," with Theodore Friedmann as Chair
(Friedmann is the Director of the Gene Therapy Lab at the University of
California San Diego), and Professor Lee Sweeney (Professor and Chairman
of Physiology, University of Pennsylvania) as one of its members (see below
for the role of Professor Lee Sweney on research on insulin-like growth factor
1 and the so-called "Schwarzenegger mice").

While it may sound surprising, WADA has included gene transfer technologies in the Prohibited List since 2003, under the umbrella of "gene doping." The very act of labelling this type of genetic modification as "doping"
is a significant act, clearly connoting an official negative attitude towards the
practice. But can gene transfer techniques be classified as doping? Before addressing this question, we need to understand – adopting a similar strategy as
the one adopted in the previous chapters – what we are talking about when
we talk about gene enhancement from a scientific point of view, distinguishing scientifically feasible from fictional scenarios. This should be the first and
foremost responsibility of all bioethicists involved in the discussions around
gene doping, as highlighted by Atry and co-authors (2011). Only afterwards
can we analyse whether, and on what basis, gene transfer technologies for
enhancement purposes can count as doping.

---

1   http://www.wada-ama.org/en/Science-Medicine/Science-topics/Gene-Dop-
     ing/ [Accessed, March 18, 2014]

The Targets of Gene Enhancement

Gene transfer aimed at enhancing athletic performance (hence gene enhancement, or GE) employs the same techniques used in gene transfer for therapeutic purposes, which is referred to as gene therapy (GT). Gene transfer is based on the delivery to a cell of a gene through a carrier (usually a modified virus, but also a liposomic particle, or no carrier at all), with the aim of compensating an absent or abnormally functioning gene in GT, and with the purpose of reinforcing muscular systems, increasing the number of red cells, or increasing the threshold for pain in GE, as discussed in detail below. Gene transfer differs from other more traditional modes of doping insofar as, instead of administering the doping substance (e.g. erythropoietin, or EPO) to the athlete exogenously, a gene is administered to the body via a carrier, so that the body itself will produce EPO in higher quantities.

The following are some of the most plausible targets for gene enhancement:

- Growth hormone (GH): has a multitude of effects on the body associated with growth, including a well-documented stimulatory effect on carbohydrate and fatty acid metabolism, and a possible anabolic effect on muscle proteins. To note that recombinant GH is already being used as a doping agent in sports. (Baumann 2012)
- Insulin growth factor 1 (IGF-1): stimulates cellular proliferation, somatic growth and differentiation. In 1998, Dr Lee Sweeney (to note, now a member of WADA Gene Doping Expert Group) was the first to conduct in vivo gene transfer studies in mice using IGF-1. (Barton-Davis et al. 1998) The gene transfer successfully increased the strength of the mice, leading the press to dub them as "Schwarzenegger mice." (Bartlett 2003) Macedo and co-authors created a mouse model of gene enhancement based on the AAV-mediated delivery of the IGF-1 cDNA to multiple muscles. (Macedo et al. 2012) This treatment determined marked muscle hypertrophy, neovascularization and fast-to-slow fibre type transition, similar to what happens to athletes during endurance training. In functional terms, IGF-1 transferred mice showed impressive endurance gain, as determined by an exhaustive swimming test. The authors warn against the potential misuses of AAV-IGF1 as a "realistic way to achieve a greater athletic performance." (Macedo et al. 2012)

- Myostatin: is a protein that acts as a negative regulator of muscle mass. Mice in which the myostatin gene has been inactivated show marked muscle hypertrophy (Li et al. 2010) and a recent report described similar muscle hypertrophy in a child carrying mutations in both copies of the myostatin gene. (McFarlane et al. 2011) Therefore, blockade of myostatin action has the potential to allow athletes to rapidly increase muscle mass.
- Erythropoietin (EPO): is a glycoprotein produced by the kidney in response to a low oxygen concentration. EPO expression leads to an increase in red blood cell production and hence an increase in the blood's oxygen carrying capacity. EPO is one of the most widely used doping agents. (Leuenberger, Reichel, and Lasne 2012)
- Vascular Endothelial Growth Factor (VEGF) and other angiogenic factors: their expression improves microcirculation in muscle and hence increases oxygen and nutrient supply as well as removal of waste products. (Wells 2008) There are already clinical trials underway or completed employing gene transfer techniques for angiogenesis purposes following an ischemia (peripheral or heart) (http://clinicaltrials.gov/). In a paper co-authored with Mike McNamee and included in this work in a slightly revised form in next section, we analyse one of these clinical trials employing VEGF and investigate its permissibility from an ethical point of view in a research and in a professional sport context. (Camporesi and McNamee 2012)
- Hypoxia-inducible factor 1 alpha (HIF-1-alpha): transcription factor activated under conditions of endurance exercise and muscle hypoxia: induces both the endogenous expression of EPO and VEGF. Consequently, increased expression of HIF-1-alpha has the potential to substantially improve oxygen delivery to the skeletal and cardiac muscles. (Borrione et al. 2008)
- Peroxisome-proliferator-activated receptor gamma (PPAR-gamma): the expression of the activated form of this protein in skeletal muscle increases the running endurance of transgenic mice to double that of wild-type littermates. Gene transfer of PPAR-gamma in athletes may improve endurance capacity by increasing the proportion of oxidative slow twitch fibres. (Østergård et al. 2005)

The Repoxygen case

The first documented case of gene transfer aimed at enhancing athletic performance dates back to 2006 in Germany. Thomas Springstein, track & field coach, was found guilty of trying to procure a gene transfer product called Repoxygen to administer to supposedly oblivious athletes. Repoxygen was a viral delivery vector carrying the human EPO gene under the control of a hypoxia response element, based on the principle of increasing the number of red cells in the athlete, consequently increasing the cellular oxygen carrying capacity. (G. Reynolds 2007; Fantz 2010) Repoxygen was also an example of a direct bench to track & field transfer of technology (without passing through the bedside and the clinical trials step), as in 2006 it was in pre-clinical animal studies for a company called Oxford Biomedica. Therefore, at that time, there were no data at all on the effects and possible risks of the use of gene transfer for EPO in humans.

As it will be evident now, even though gene doping had been included under the WADA Prohibited List since 2003, it is only since 2006 and the Repoxygen case in Germany that gene enhancement has become a documented reality. Meanwhile, WADA has actively been building a confident narrative on the possibility of detecting gene doping through "sheer good-will" and generous funds[2]. Indeed, foreseeing a massive use of gene enhancement techniques in the London 2012 Olympics, WADA invested nearly $15 million to support research laboratories to develop methods for gene doping detection since its first investment in 2002. (Daiji World 2013) The funded laboratories include the Molecular Medicine-Gene Therapy laboratory at the International Centre for Genetic Engineering and Biotechnology, which received WADA funding to develop mouse models of genetic enhancement, as the one mentioned above. (Macedo, 2011) In London, the King's College Drug Control Centre directed by Dan Cowan was appointed by WADA as the only laboratory in the UK responsible for gene doping detection and for "championing Olympic integrity." (Reynolds 2012) King's College London then partnered with

---

2   The full list of up-to-date WADA-funded research projects can be found here:
     http://www.wada-ama.org/en/science-medicine/research/funded-research-
     projects/ [Accessed, July 18, 2014]

GlaxoSmithKline (GSK) to enable its world-renowned Drug Control Centre to operate a WADA accredited satellite laboratory during the London 2012 Olympic and Paralympic Games. (E. Reynolds 2012)

In 2010, WADA Director David Howman reported to the Telegraph that he was quite confident that gene enhancement strategies would be able to be detected, (Telegraph Staff 2010), but his optimism seems unjustified for reasons explained below.

Challenges to detection

Gene transfer techniques pose several unique challenges to detection. (Baoutina et al. 2008) To start with, the protein produced through gene transfer will not be different in sequence or structure from the endogenously produced one. Anti-doping techniques aimed at identifying the "markers" of the viral vectors deployed have low probability of success, as the viral vectors may be measurable only shortly after administration, lowering therefore the probabilities of discovering their presence. In addition, detection would require repeated tissue sampling, as the administration of the vector would be performed directly into the muscular target tissue. Obviously, muscle biopsies would not be a feasible option for the athlete, therefore excluding this mode of detection. (Baoutina et al. 2008) Alternative modes of detection called "transcriptional profiling" aimed at detecting changes in protein levels (compared to the physiologically measured basal level of the athlete) would require simultaneous and repeated measuring of around 1,000 proteins. (Rupert 2009)

The London 2012 Olympics did not witness those scandals of "gene doping." There were, though, gene doping speculations on Chinese swimmer Ye Shiwen, who won the mixed 400 meters setting a new world record in 4'28" and swimming the last 100 meters faster than the male US swimmer and gold medallist Ryan Lochte. This detail led to the public accusation by John Leonard, executive director of the World Swimming Coaches Association (US office), that her victory was "disturbing" , and that she may have "gene-doped." (Naish 2012) This episode calls to mind a parallel with the case of South African runner Caster Semenya, whose gold medal at the Berlin World Track & Field Championship in 2009 was also deemed "disturbing" because it was on par with male athlete performances, leading to accusations of cheating. (Discussed in Camporesi & Maugeri 2010). The British tabloid Daily Mail pounced on the Shiwen case and conjectured on the possibility of genetic modification (from Naish 2012):

> The astonishing suggestion seems to be that London 2012 may be the first Olympics in which competitors are attempting to cheat by altering their genes to build muscle and sinew, and boost their blood's oxygen-carrying powers.

Shiwen later tested negative at the anti-doping control, and John Leonard had to deliver a public apology. The result of the anti-doping control did not quench completely, though, the speculations that China may have undertaken state-sponsored genetic modification experiments to breed athletes. This scenario is not too far from documented Chinese-based boot-camps for very young children where traditional modes of talent-scouting have been coupled with new genetic technologies (see sections 3.3 and 3.4).

Risks for the health of the athlete

Gene enhancement techniques pose several risks to the health of the athlete that relate both to the kind of vector used (usually a modified virus), and to the encoded transgene. (Harridge and Velloso 2008) As to the former, while gene transfer has proven *relatively safe* in clinical trials so far (with some major exceptions, such as the death of 18-year old clinical trial subject Jess Gelsinger due to immunoshock to the viral vector in 1998), (Lehrman 1999; Hollon 2000) it is plausible to infer that gene enhancement, since outlawed, would be carried out in laboratories with less stringent regulations, therefore posing even more health hazards. Gene enhancement represents indeed one perfect example of technological determinism as discussed by Agar (Agar 2005) and presented in section 1.4: even if we were to reach an agreement through public deliberation that gene enhancement is an ethically problematic technology, it is plausible to speculate that somewhere else in the world techniques of gene transfer aimed to enhance athletic performance would be developed. As explained at the end of chapter 1 though, this should not discourage us from tackling the issue of gene doping from an ethical point of view.

As to the latter risks relative to the encoded transgene, they are similar to the risks encountered in more traditional doping modes, but in addition both the level and the duration of protein expression are less amenable to control. For example, growth hormone and insulin-like growth factor 1 are both potent mitogen (i.e. stimulate cellular proliferation) and anti-apoptotic (i.e. inhibit physiological death mechanisms) agents, leading to an increased risk of oncogenesis. Overexpression of EPO causes an increase in haematocrit (i.e. the ratio of the volume of red blood cells to the total volume of blood), which in turn makes the blood more viscous and increases the load on the heart. Potential consequences include blockage of microcirculation, stroke and heart failure. In addition, the uncontrolled expression of the transgenes may in itself be harmful. Adenoviral vectors have been clearly associated with morbidity and in one case death after vascular administration in 1998, as mentioned above.

WADA's Definition of Gene Doping

As illustrated above, WADA has included gene enhancement techniques in the blacklist of prohibited substances since 2003. As we can read in the following statement published on WADA's official publication *Play True*, it is evident that WADA considers gene transfer technologies aimed at enhancing athletic performance as a form of doping:

> Gene doping represents a threat to the integrity of sport [c] and the health of athletes [b], and as the international organization responsible for promoting, coordinating and monitoring the global fight against doping in sport in all its forms, WADA is devoting significant resources and attention to ways that will enable the detection of gene doping. (WADA Official Publication *Play True* 2008)

As mentioned above, two of the three criteria are currently sufficient for inclusion of a substance in the Prohibited List.[3] The most recent version of the

---

3   WADA is now in the process of revising its Code, expected to come into effect with a new version in 2015. (For a discussion, see Camporesi and McNamee 2014)

Prohibited List contains the following definition for Gene Doping:

> The following, with the potential to enhance sport performance, are
> prohibited:
> 1. The transfer of polymers of nucleic acids or nucleic acid analogues;
> 2. The use of normal or genetically modified cells.

Gene doping is therefore defined by WADA to include the non-therapeutic use of genes, genetic elements, or cells that have the potential to enhance athletic performance. Note that this is a very broad definition that encompasses both gene and cellular therapy, and by choosing to adopt such a broad definition WADA aims to ensure that all possibilities of gene or cellular transfer aimed at enhancing athletic performance are covered under the wide umbrella of "gene doping." In the second issue of *Play True*, WADA spokesperson and Chair of the expert group on Gene Doping, Professor Theodore Friedmann, explains why gene doping is unethical:

> This technology is highly experimental and completely inappropriate where
> the goal might be something other than the cure of life-threatening disease
> like cancer, neurological degenerations and so on. To apply this very imma-
> ture technology to athletes or to any young, healthy people for the purpose
> of increasing some already-normal function, in my mind, is unethical and
> constitutes deliberate professional malpractice. (WADA Official Publication
> *Play True* 2007)

Note that Friedmann's concern about gene doping is merely a concern on the safety of the athletes, and while the concern for safety may make, at the present state of knowledge, a persuasive case to prohibit the use of gene modification in sports at a later point in time, this does not seem to constitute sufficient ground to ban it. The most important question, which I will address below, is whether genetic modification would still be ethically unacceptable in conditions where the technology were sufficiently safe. I will therefore examine and unpack WADA's position regarding doping, and discuss whether it can be applied to gene transfer technologies, focusing my analysis on the third criterion for inclusion of a substance in the Prohibited List, i.e., the "spirit of sport."

Infringing the "spirit" of sport?

What is it to talk about the "spirit of sport"? Murray defines sport as "the paramount public expression of our embodied humanness" and argues that the achievement of excellence in athletic performance requires a combination of both physical natural talents and of character traits such as "perseverance, dedication, and a willingness to suffer in pursuit of a valued goal." (Murray 2009a) Catlin and Murray write that the spirit of sport is about winning "with the best combination of natural ability, stamina, courage, willingness to undergo intense and difficult training, and strategic cunning." (Catlin and Murray 1996) In 2008's second issue of *Play True*, Murray writes:

> We need to go back again to a key question: What is sport about? What contributes to its beauty and its value? What gives sport its meaning? I don't want my children or grandchildren to have to go through genetic enhancement to compete on a level playing field. ... we can do with the natural talents we have, perfecting them through human excellence, persistent effort and dedication, and not with artificial enhancement and engineering. (WADA Official Publication *Play True* 2008)

Sigmund Loland points out that the prospect of gene transfer for enhancement purposes is so disturbing for sports ethics because it forces us to acknowledge that the "natural lottery" of genetics is increasingly getting less random as our knowledge of human genetics expands. Writes Loland: "It is an individual's genetic predisposition to develop phenotypes of relevance to performance in the sport in question. The distribution of talent in the natural lottery is a random process." (Loland 2002, 69) In this sense, gene transfer would challenge the spirit of sport as defined by Murray as above, because genetic interventions would undermine the very ability of sport to distinguish those who passively inherit their talents from their progenitors, from those who actively acquired them from their physicians, or through some other external means. Michael Sandel also wrote on genetic enhancement as corrupting the spirit of sport:

The real problem with genetically altered athletes is that they corrupt athletic competition as a human activity that honors the cultivation as display of natural talents. (Sandel 2004, 55)

Implicit in Murray's and Sandel's statements and in WADA's definition of doping there is a deeply value-laden interpretation of sport, comprising an "intrinsic value" or an "essence" of Olympism. Neither WADA nor its spokespersons, though, attempt to spell out what this essence is. This is what the WADA Code says in regard to the mission of preserving the "spirit of sport":

Anti-doping programs seek to preserve what is intrinsically valuable about sport. This intrinsic value is often referred to as the "spirit of sport," it is the essence of Olympism; [it] is characterized by the following values: ethics, fair play and honesty, health, excellence in performance, character and education, fun and joy, teamwork, dedication and commitment, respect for rule and laws, respect for self and other participants, courage, community and solidarity. Doping is fundamentally contrary to the spirit of sport. (WADA Code 2012)

But the explanation of what these values amount to and of why certain kinds of enhancement actually threaten them is missing. As argued extensively in Camporesi and Maugeri (2011)[4], while an appropriate analysis of the ethical justifiability of genetic enhancement in sports must take into account an analysis of the values of sports, the assumption of "essentialism" in sports seems to be unwarranted.

Indeed, professional sport is highly technological, as athletes nowadays are able to improve their performances with a larger array of aids than in the past. Talk of purity of sports overlooks that all elite sports are both "play and display," i.e., they thrive both on "internal goods" after MacIntyre (MacIntyre 1984) (such values as commitment, channelled concentration, controlled aggression and power, courage in the face of suffering, dedication, strategic intensity, tenacity, to name but a few of the virtues of sports), and on external

---

4   Partly included in this work in section 4.4.

goods or rewards, as the achievement of considerable esteem, glory, honour, and wealth. (McNamee 2008). It is also important to note how the norms that govern sports are highly heterogeneous. Therefore, when evaluating the impact of gene enhancement on athletic performance, we should ask ourselves to what extent, if any, genetic technologies enhance or diminish our admiration for human athletic achievements, in relation to a particular sport.

As argued by Tom Douglas (2007), the case for restricting enhancement is stronger in sports than outside sports, due to the different values intrinsic in the practice of sports and in other practices. This distinction depends on how genetic technologies affect the way in which we admire elite athletes and their achievements. Douglas spells out two main models for what it is that that we admire most in elite athletes, namely the "Athenian" model, where the value and meaning of sports lies in revealing the natural potential of athletes; and the "effort" model, where the value and meaning of sports lies in rewarding and praising athletes for their hard work and effort.

The adoption of the Athenian model only though seems unrealistic, as we normally allow all kinds of external edges to enhance the natural potential, i.e., training/equipment/facilities (eye and knee surgery, training in hyperbaric rooms, and so on). But a position based only on effort does not correspond either to how we normally value and perceive sports, as we do not praise or admire professional athletes only for 'trying hard' without succeeding. Neither of the two models, taken alone, can be a plausible account of what we value in sports. A more realistic view is one that combines the two and holds that the outcomes of sport should be determined by natural ability and effort, and that we value sport because it serves as a test of these two characteristics. For these reasons, I think that a better approach to define the ethical permissibility of a gene enhancement technology is the following, which reflects on how a technology affects a sports practice in a contextualized way:

Cooper defines technology as a "human-made means to serve human interests and goals." (Cooper 1995) Elaborating on Cooper's definition, Loland defines sports technology as a human-made means to serve human interests and goals in or related to sport. (Loland 2009) Murray, when evaluating the role of a technology in sports, outlines three possible outcomes in relation to an ethical standard (Murray 2009a, 157–9):

A technology may be ethically desirable: insofar as it may, for example, reduce the impact of factors other than natural talents and their virtuous perfection by reducing unequal access to the legitimate means of enhancing performance. Example: hypoxic chamber (levelling the playing field for athletes who because of geography or lack of money, cannot "live high, train low").

A technology may be ethically permissible: they are ethically "neutral" in respect to the relation between talent, virtue and performance. For example, inequalities of access to superb coaching and training facilities are very pervasive. Normally the differential access of athletes due to their geographical and economical conditions to different degrees of coaching and of training facilities is regarded as a tolerable inequality, a status quo.

A technology may be ethically prohibited: this should be the case when it undermines the meaning of sport by interfering significantly with the relationship between natural talents, their virtuous perfection, and athletic success. Examples: blood doping, EPO.

The question then becomes: In which of the above categories can we find genetic enhancements? I argue that is a matter of context, and of spelling out the values intrinsic in the practice under scrutiny. In the following section I consider one of the latest applications of biomedical innovation applied directly from the bench to track & field, namely the use of gene transfer to increase circulation and tolerance to pain in patients and in athletes engaged in endurance races.

3.2 Gene transfer for pain: A tool to cope with the intractable, or an unethical endurance-enhancing technology?

We consider here[5] two plausible scenarios in which an individual is seeking treatment with gene transfer tools to cope better with pain. In the first sce-

---

5   This section first appeared in a slightly different form in *Life Sciences, Society and Policy Journal* (2012):8(1):20-31 with title "Gene Transfer for Pain: A tool to cope with the intractable, or an unethical endurance-enhancing technology?," co-authored with Mike McNamee.

nario the individual is a patient; in the second an athlete. The general question explored here is whether it is ethically justifiable for the individual to seek an experimental gene transfer treatment in order to raise her tolerance to pain. We employ here a comparative strategy to highlight the similarities and dissimilarities between the ethical frameworks used to evaluate the two scenarios, and to reach conclusions regarding the justifiability of the potential practice.

Untreatable pain represents an enormous problem to society. As estimated by current statistics, approximately 20 per cent of the adult population suffers from chronic pain, and the financial cost to society is estimated at more than €200 billion per annum in Europe, and $150 billion per annum in the US. (Tracey and Bushnell 2009) Treatment options are limited, with many patients either not responding or having incomplete pain reduction. (Breivik et al. 2006) In the last decade, several translational clinical trials have been carried out that employed gene transfer tools to try to overcome this medical need. Gene transfer trials certainly qualify as translational trials, as they are designed to bring to the bedside the tools developed at the bench of a molecular biology laboratory. A search performed with keywords "gene transfer" and "pain" on the National Health Institutes clinical trials revealed 20 clinical trials that are either completed or in recruitment. (Clinicaltrials.gov 2014a) To date eleven clinical trials have been completed. (Clinicaltrials.gov 2014a) Some of these trials are aimed at treating intractable cancer pain, some at treating pain associated with angina pectoris, others at epidermolysis bullosa (a heritable condition where connective tissue disease causes painful blisters in the skin and mucosal membranes), and others to treat the pain associated with peripheral arterial occlusion (a mini-stroke in the leg which causes the necrosis of muscular tissue leading to impaired functionality and chronic pain). This last kind of pain, and the related clinical trial, serves as a case study for our comparative evaluation between a medical context and a sports context, where the former is a traditionally conceived therapeutic intervention, and the latter is one where the intervention rests in the grey zone between therapy and enhancement – or as it has been labelled, therapeutic enhancement. (Tannsjo 2010) We set out the two scenarios below and evaluate them ethically according to two different frameworks.

Scenario (a): The Patient

In scenario (a), the protagonist of the US TV series Dr Gregory House, suffered from peripheral ischemia to a leg, which left him limping and with intractable chronic pain, due to the extensive necrotic muscular tissue in his thigh muscles. He is seeking an alternative solution in a gene transfer clinical trial. Dr House can perhaps be seen as a contemporary instance of the archetypical mythological figure of the "wounded healer" Chiron, who is able to heal others but unable to heal himself. After having tried many standard and less standard treatments unsuccessfully, our protagonist is now seeking experimental treatments, i.e. treatments that are currently being tested in clinical trials and not yet approved by national regulatory bodies such as the US Food & Drug Administration (FDA) or the European Medicines Agency (EMA), and are unavailable on the market. Among the gene transfer trials currently active or recruiting, one study stands out as the perfect match for a patient like Gregory House. The trial (Identifier # NCT00304837) is a Phase 1 study that seeks to transfer the DNA codifying for Vascular Endothelial Growth Factor (VEGF) in the legs of patients with peripheral artery disease (PAD). (Clinicaltrials.gov 2014b) PAD encompasses a range of conditions presenting with blockages in the arteries in the limbs. The nature of the disease is progressive, so that it frequently leads to patients presenting with claudication (i.e. limping) or critical limb ischemia (CLI). (Mughal et al. 2012) It is this former manifestation of PAD that I will discuss in what follows. Most Phase 1 studies are aimed at testing the safety of a new pharmaceutical or treatment in a restricted number of patients, after the treatment has proved efficacious in laboratory testing and animal models, but some – like this one – may also test the efficacy of the agent under study. According to the trial protocol, the DNA codifying for the VEGF protein is injected into the affected legs of the trial subjects on three separate occasions, each two weeks apart. The DNA codifier then directs the cells of the artery wall to increase production of VEGF, which has been shown to cause new blood vessels to grow around the blockages in the leg arteries. (Mughal et al. 2012) It has also been demonstrated that increased VEGF expression through gene transfer techniques improves microcirculation in muscle, and hence increased oxygen and nutrient supply, as well as removal of waste products. (Giacca and Zacchigna 2012) Kim et al. have observed evidence of growth of new collateral vessels, relief of ischemic pain and ulcer healing in patients with CLI. (Kim et al. 2004) The NCT00304837 trial aims not only at testing the safety of VEGF-gene transfer, but also at improving rest pain and/or healing the ulcers caused by PAD. (Clinicaltrials.gov 2013b) Generally speaking, safety concerns about gene transfer are related both to the kind of carrier/vector being used (usually a modified virus) and to the encoded transgene. In this case study, the former are eliminated by injecting the DNA coding for the VEGF protein directly into the patients' leg muscles, without any viral or non-viral carrier, thus eliminating the risks inherent in the vectors and common to many other gene transfer trials. As to the latter risks, it has been shown that overexpression of VEGF causes haemangiomas (benign tumours characterised by an increased number of normal or abnormal vessels filled with blood) in skeletal muscle in mouse animal models. (Springer et al. 1998) In addition, angiogenesis can have detrimental consequences in non-target tissues. In particular, it can facilitate tumour vascularization (and therefore, increased growth) or plaque angiogenesis in non-target tissues. (Baumgartner 2000) Transient peripheral edema (swelling) due to increased local perfusion is a relatively common and mild side effect. More serious adverse effects have rarely been observed and are mostly related to the use of viral vectors, therefore are not pertinent to this trial where DNA is injected in the form of a plasmid (a circular molecule of DNA). (Muona et al. 2012) A recent study conducted by Muona and co-authors and aimed at assessing the long-term side effects (10+years) of local VEGF gene transfer to ischemic lower limbs found that adenovirus or plasmid or liposome mediated intravascular local gene transfer does not increase the risk of malignancies, diabetes or any other disease in the long term. The authors also identified as a key element to safe gene transfer the local delivery, which reduced the risk of systematic spread of the vector, as well of adverse side-effects to other organs. This suggests that the technique described here could be safely applied both in trial subjects and in healthy individuals (which is pertinent to Scenario (b), below).

As noted by Mughal et al., PAD cannot be attributed to one specific genetic cause, and greater therapeutic efficacy could be obtained by targeted gene transfer using multiple growth factors. (Mughal et al. 2012) Indeed, angiogenic gene transfer strategies such as VEGF gene transfer are by no means the only ones being explored in the treatment of chronic pain, (Goins, Cohen, and Glorioso 2012) but appear to be among the most advanced in terms of clinical development, while other strategies are still at the pre-clinical level (animal studies). While a certain degree of speculation is necessary in this thought experiment, there seems to be sufficient scientific and medical evidence to argue that gene transfer for pain has very plausible applications for enhancing athletic performances.

Scenario (b): The elite athlete

In scenario (b), the would-be protagonist is an elite athlete competing in an endurance event, such as cross-country skiing, marathon running, tour cycling, triathlon, or another event of similar extended duration. This hypothetical elite athlete is seeking VEGF-gene transfer for two reasons: a) to cope better with the pain inherent in the event, and b) to perform better and gain a competitive advantage. The growth of blood vessels in the limbs, as demonstrated by the clinical trial described above, is likely to aid the athlete in her performance by increasing the oxygen-carrying capacity to the limbs (nutrient supply) and the removal of waste products. It is also obvious that an athlete feeling less pain could perform better, *ceteribus paribus*, than other athletes experiencing a greater degree of pain.

Comparing the scenarios

How are we to understand the similarities and differences between these two scenarios, and to what extent will the context determine whether it is ethically justifiable for an individual to seek an experimental gene transfer treatment to cope better with pain? To what extent is the ethical permissibility of the practice dependent upon the context of gene transfer? We respond to these questions by spelling out two ethical frameworks that might be adopted in order to analyse the two scenarios.

Scenario (a): Ethics of translational research

We do not normally regard pain as an essential or valuable part of our lives. On the contrary, we take measures to diminish or if possible eliminate pain from our daily lives, and from the lives of those who are dear to us. Even in illnesses where pain is present, we try to eliminate it, although it may not be possible to cure the patient of the underlying cause. Palliative care, which we consider an essential part of treating a sick human being with dignity, is predicated on such an understanding.

The first framework we use to analyse the scenarios is (a) is the "ethics of translational research" approach recently developed by Jonathan Kimmelman. (Kimmelman 2010) Kimmelman develops the concept of 'translational distance,' which refers to the space created between cutting-edge biomedical research, and clinical applications. This new concept is necessary as it is not possible to apply the concept of "clinical equipoise," as defined by Freedman as "a state of honest, professional disagreement in the community of experts about the preferred treatment," (Freedman 1987) to translational trials such as gene transfer trials. This happens because the level of uncertainty is so high in first-in-human research employing gene transfer techniques that the robust epistemic thresholds required for clinical equipoise cannot be secured. In its place, the concept of translational distance is a useful and insightful kind of "epistemic heuristics" to understand the bidirectional flow of knowledge between the bench and the bedside. While traditionally the value of early clinical trials has been regarded only in terms of their "progressive value" towards later Phase 2 and Phase 3 studies, in Kimmelman's model Phase 1 translational studies have a "bidirectional, non -progressive" epistemic value if they stimulate preclinical research or if they stimulate further clinical development. In addition, adopting a translational distance model with a non-progressive epistemic value for these trials would help to dispel the "therapeutic misconception" (Henderson et al. 2006; Horng and Grady 2003) which is a widespread phenomenon among (often desperate) Phase I clinical trials participants. Therapeutic misconception arises when subjects misinterpret the primary purpose of a clinical trial as therapeutic, and conflate the goals of research with the goals of clinical care. As shown in a study of consent documents of gene transfer clinical trials, 20 per cent of consent documents for gene transfer trials fail to explain their purpose as establishing safety and dosage, while only 41 per cent of oncology trials identify palliative care as an alternative to participation. Moreover, the term gene therapy is used with twice the frequency of the term gene transfer. (Kimmelman and

Levenstadt 2005) As defined by Kimmelman, the concept of translational distance "is intended to prompt researchers, review committees, and policy-makers to contemplate the size of the 'inferential gap' separating completed preclinical studies and projected human trial results," (Kimmelman 2010, 118) and should inform both the design of the studies (that need to incorporate endpoints that make it possible for the knowledge produced to have an impact in terms of further research), and the ethical approval of the trial. This needs to take into account the concept of translational distance rather than that of clinical equipoise, as the former better captures the reality of how information flows in translational research. As for the individual seeking to be enrolled in such an experimental trial, we recommend that researchers spell out the potential risks and benefits of the experimental procedure to the would-be volunteer. Researchers should also evaluate the severity of the pre-existing condition in the subject and its refractoriness to other standard treatments; and they should evaluate the subject's decisional autonomy, which will be predicated on reasonable comprehension (and voluntariness) in relation to the foregoing.

Returning to our fictional protagonist, we can see that in this particular case the risks inherent in gene transfer trials due to the viral vectors are eliminated by injecting VEGF directly into the leg muscles of the patients, and therefore the translational distance between the bench and the bedside can also be considered a modest "inferential gap." In addition, the pre-existing condition of chronic pain caused by peripheral artery ischemia is severe and refractory to standard treatment. Finally, Dr Gregory House seems to be in a position to make an autonomous decision, one that is not clouded by thera-peutic misconception. As autonomy plays a fundamental role in the ethical framework describing the medical context, there would need to be strong rea-sons to justify interference with the patient's self-regarding and autonomous choice to participate in the trial, even recognising – as we do – that the patient may have no available option (apart from palliative care) other than participat-ing in the trial, due to the severity of his condition and the unavailability of therapeutic alternatives. Provided that all the above conditions were met, we might reasonably conclude that his informed consent to participating in the VEGF-clinical trial would be valid.

Scenario (b): Ethics of sports enhancement

How should we frame the request of an athlete seeking VEGF-gene transfer for the purposes of better coping with pain during a competition? In the first instance, her participation might look like a case of what we could call "physician-assisted doping." As already mentioned, the World Anti-Doping Agency (WADA) sets out three criteria used in the decision to call a product or process "doping." (WADA Code 2012) These pertain to (i) the (potential) performance-enhancing effects; (ii) the potential harm to health; the (potential) health risks. Only two criteria need apply for a product or process to be prohibited. The Anti-Doping Code recognises the rights of athletes to secure healthcare, and that this right supersedes anti-doping regulations. This does not, however, allow the patient-athlete *carte blanche*. Prior to utilising banned products or processes athletes on a registered testing pool (who are on notice that they may be randomly tested) must submit a Therapeutic Use Exemption (TUE) Certificate signed by a relevant medical authority. This certifies that the therapy is necessary for the athlete's condition and that no nondoping alternative is available. Clearly, the process is open to abuse. Leaving aside for the present the added complexities of unethical behaviour, let us assume that our athlete is asking for a TUE from the relevant authority. In addition to the World Anti-Doping Agency, this might be an International Federation, such as the International Association of Athletics Federations (IAAF), or an event organiser such as the International Olympic Committee (IOC) or the International Paralympic Committee, who (interestingly) take exclusive charge of in-competition testing during the Olympic and Paralympic Games. There is very little to suggest that a TUE would be achievable in this scenario. Despite TUE precedents for beta-blockers in relation to cardiac patient-athletes in target-accuracy events (such as archery), it is highly unlikely that a TUE would be given for mere pain relief where that pain is simply a marker for injury (and where there may be performance enhancement side effects). The deputy director of the World Anti Doping Laboratory in Cologne, widely recognised as one of the premier testing laboratories, recently remarked upon the practice of using analgesics as analogous to doping:

It is a grey zone. In my opinion pain killers fulfil all requirements of a doping substance because normally pain is a protection mechanism of the body
and with pain killers you switch off this protection system. (McGrath 2012)

Given the longstanding routine use and abuse of painkillers in elite sport,
(Huizenga 1995; Nixon 1992; Nixon 1993) it might be argued that the introduction of VEGF would represent merely an extension of everyday practice.
In both scenarios analyzed here, consideration would have to be given to the
autonomy of the decision-making of the individual in reaching an ethically
justifiable intervention. While in the second scenario, this could be deemed a
necessary condition, in the first scenario it might be considered both a necessary and sufficient condition, provided that the conditions for a modest
translational distance were met, as they are in our case study. Why then can
an autonomous decision not be regarded as a necessary and sufficient condition also in the context of elite sports? Well, in addition to determining the
conditions of consent, additional factors regarding the ethical permissibility
of VEGF-gene transfer in an athletic context must be considered:

In contrast to scenario (a), pain can be seen as an essential, integral part
of endurance sports. Performing at an elite level in endurance sport and not
experiencing pain are mutually exclusive. Indeed, an athlete's ability to tolerate
pain is one of the fundamental characteristics that determine athletic performance and provide an advantage in competition. Lance Armstrong famously
referred to the Tour de France as "an exercise in pointless suffering."(Fry
2006) He and others have talked insightfully about wanting to take opponents
(metaphorically) to places that they could not endure. (Hamilton 2012) The
capacity to endure high levels of pain over significant time is a highly prized
trait in multi-day/week Tour event cycling. (Hamilton 2012) Indeed one may
refer to endurance cyclists as "communities of suffering." (McNamee 2008)
Not only is it the case that we must distinguish the experience of pain from
suffering, (Cassell 2004) in sports (Lurie 2006; McNamee 2006), but in addition there are, of course, different kinds of pain an athlete can experience in
competition. (Koessler 2006) One is the acute kind that can be defined as an
intense and specific pain that occurs suddenly, frequently a result of injury, and
often experienced by athletes competing in football or other contact sports.

Moreover, one can experience such pain in endurance events too – the cycle crash, the herniated disc in running, and so on. VEGF-gene transfer treatment would be meaningless for this kind of pain, so it is irrelevant to this discussion. Rather, we wish to discuss the kind of pain that occurs during endurance exercise. This may include muscle soreness or a burning sensation in the lungs, the feeling that one's heart will explode if the same level of intense effort is maintained much longer, and so forth. The strength of these sensations can range from unpleasant to what is typically thought of as unbearable pain. This second kind of pain is typical of endurance sports such as marathons, triathlon, long distance swimming and cycling, cross-country skiing, and so on. Among athletes, the former kind of pain is often referred to as a "bad" kind, as it impairs the ability of the athlete to continue playing or competing, while the latter is referred to as a "good" kind of pain, as it pushes the athlete to compete and perform at a higher level. Indeed, many athletes regard this second or "good kind" of pain as an achievement, and as an essential part of their life and identity as elite athletes. (Howe 2004)

The level of physical training of an athlete can raise the level of pain that he/she is able to endure, and make a difference in his/her performance. Athletes also report that the level of their "mental toughness" (Crust 2007; Gucciardi, Gordon, and Dimmock 2009) makes a difference in their ability to cope with pain. Different individuals, though, start from very different baselines in their abilities to endure pain, (Dolgin 2010) and this is one of the factors, among many other biological and environmental factors, that affect an athlete's performance. Among these are: their birth place (contrast pre-athletic life at altitude, and how this affects phenotypic factors, with competitors born at or near sea level); wealth and other non-athletic factors that can enhance the possibilities of success (contrast athletes or teams with and without sports psychological services, or sponsorships that improve equipment access), genetic conditions that may confer an advantage over fellow athletes by increasing the amount of erythrocytes and oxygen supply to muscle cells (consider for example the case of Finnish skier Eero Mäntyranta who won two gold medals in cross-country skiing at the 1964 Winter Olympics). It was later discovered that he had primary familial and congenital polycythemia (PFCP), which causes an increase in red blood cell mass and haemoglobin due to a mutation in the erythropoietin receptor (EPOR) gene. (Tannsjo 2005; Epstein 2013)

There is no absolutely agreed upon standard or trigger as to when sports administrators or regulatory bodies like WADA try to even out genetic and biological differences to reach a sufficiently "level playing field" for all athletes: some inequalities are systematically excluded, while others are ignored. (Loland 2002) What happens in practice is that we do not usually try to level out biological and genetic factors affecting athletic performance, even where we know that those factors confer an advantage (as with Mäntyranta), although there has been a lively debate about new IAAF and IOC rules which exclude women athletes with hyperandrogenism from competing in women's events on the basis of a supposed unfair advantage derived from increased levels of testosterone. (Camporesi and Maugeri 2010; Karkazis et al. 2012) Typically, philosophers generally agree that the question centres around notions of fairness and equal opportunity, or what Loland calls Fair Opportunity Principle. (Loland 2009)

Let us think counter-factually here: if we were to try to equalise all the starting conditions (of which tolerance to pain is, again, merely one example) we would move in the direction of having all athletes crossing the finish line at the same point, and then what would be left of the meaning of sport and athletic performance? After all we are precisely interested in distinguishing among excellent performers and performances. Only in certain circumstances, such as horse racing, do sports institutions initiate handicapping systems. And this, it might reasonably be argued, is to keep the competition tight and promote gambling interests. In other scenarios, where a league system – heavily underwritten by commercial media interests – has an incentive to prolong interests and more broadly spread opportunities to win, we find systems like the lower teams gaining access to the best new potential players in a draft system (such as in American Football). But in the main, we would not normally level out the effects of the genetic lottery in sports. If an athlete is 1 metre 40 we steer them away from high jump. If they are 2 metres tall, we do not encourage them to pursue a career as a professional jockey, and so on.

As mentioned above, different athletes have different baselines and different abilities to cope with pain. While we do try to give people tools better to cope with pain in everyday life, where pain is not seen to be an essential or meaningful part of the activity we are performing, in the elite-sports context we do not give people those tools, because pain, as described above, is a fundamental part of practising and competing at an elite level. Pain can be distinguished from non-relevant inequalities, as for example the kind of shoes or swimsuits or bikes the athletes run, swim or cycle with, which do not impact upon the mental and physical qualities that are the source of our admiration for athletes and which are instrumental to the securing of victory. For these sorts of products, however, we can and do insist upon degrees of standardisation. Thus, in baseball, cricket, or tennis there are regulations regarding the size and composition of the striking implement and the ball. Curiously, in Formula 1 racing there are prizes for both the best driver and the best constructors: the best supporting team of engineers and technologists. But even here there are strict rules about engineering variations. In European football, there are even suggestions that there should be financial fair play, so that team owners cannot "buy" victory by purchasing sufficiently large numbers of the talent pool. We cannot, however, "level-out" the capacity for enduring pain in endurance events without usurping or compromising a key psychological variable inherent within the test. By levelling the ability to endure pain, we would also diminish a substantial part of the meaning of athletic performance, which can be understood as trying to break one's own limits given the starting conditions one has. That is why the toleration of pain qualifies as a relevant inequality that serves *inter alia* to demarcate athletic merit. That is also why we consider that genetically based therapy for pain should not be permitted as it would undermine the meaning of sport by interfering significantly "with the relationship between natural talents, their virtuous perfection, and athletic success." (Murray 2009a) In other words, our view of the athlete's capacity for pain tolerance is that it should be seen as a relevant inequality and essential for the meaning of competition. In the model developed by Loland and Hoppeler that combines a biologically based approach with a Fair Opportunity principle, the use of VEGF transfer could be understood as a way to go beyond human phenotypic plasticity, and thus to go against the Fair Opportunity principle and the idea of the virtuous development of talent. (Loland and Hoppeler 2012)

To conclude, the differences between the two scenarios we have presented are many and varied. In the latter the choice is fundamentally a self-regarding one, predicated on individual autonomy together with a risk/benefits calculation as the principal factor determining the ethics of that decision. Nevertheless, in elite endurance sports contexts individual autonomy ceases to play the decisive role in the ethical analysis. Sports have traditionally incorporated paternalistic practices regarding the health of competitors but also the fairness of the structuring of competition in order to produce admirable victors. The context of gene-transfer matters for the evaluation of the ethical desirability or permissibility of the experimental practice we are analysing: while in an everyday life scenario, pain does not play a meaningful role (with some noted exceptions), pain does play a meaningful and constitutive role in endurance athletic competition, along with a range of other anatomical, physiological and psychological factors. By increasing the capacity for pain-tolerance, or even subtracting it altogether from the sports picture, we would inevitably subtract also a fundamental part of the meaning of that picture. We conclude, therefore, that while we would not interfere with the decision of Dr House to be enrolled in a trial for VEGF-gene transfer, we could not justify the request of the athlete seeking VEGF-gene transfer to increase her tolerance to pain. As a tool to cope with the intractable pain that visits afflicted patients, VEGF-gene transfer is ethically justifiable and desirable. In endurance sports, the use of VEGF-gene transfer as an endurance enhancement technology is not merely ethically unjustifiable; it compromises an element essential to the activity itself.

In the next section I consider the ethical implications of genetic technologies to identify and measure children's potentials.

3.3 Genetic technologies to scout out children's precocious talents

At first glance, the use of genetic technologies after-birth would seem to be less controversial than the use of genetic technology at the embryonic or foetal stage: after all, how much can genetic technologies really shape an already existing person? And also: do we not already grant a great degree of leeway to parents in deciding how to rear and educate their children? Parents can impose their religion, hobbies, choice of school and friends on their children, and go to great lengths to "nurture" their children's talents: from submitting them to heavy training schedules, to hiring private teachers or tutors, to sending their children to intensive summer camps, and so on. While these practices are occasionally subjected to criticisms for their strictness, it is generally accepted that parents can steer their children even aggressively in a particular direction. Not only, but we usually think that parents whose children exhibit precocious talents are bestowed with a duty to nurture them, and would not be considered to be "good parents" if they failed to do so. Michael Sandel wrote on this point:

> We usually admire parents who seek the best for their children, who spare no effort to help them achieve happiness and success. Some parents confer advantages on their children by enrolling them in expensive schools, hiring private tutors, sending them to tennis camp, providing them with piano lessons, ballet lessons, swimming lessons, SAT-prep courses,[6] and so on. If it is permissible and even admirable for parents to help their children in these ways, why isn't it equally admirable for parents to use whatever genetic technologies may emerge (provided they are safe) to enhance their children's intelligence, musical ability, or athletic prowess? (Sandel 2004, 7)

Parental attitudes like those described above by Sandel are not unique to genetic enhancements. They are, instead, new instances of old practices of child-rearing, which existed before there was any talk or discussion or enhancement. (DeGrazia 2012, 128–9) While I agree with DeGrazia that aggressive talent scouting practices are nothing new, I do not think concerns about these practices can be dismissed so easily only by references to other, established ones. Instead, the use of genetic technologies to gain a competitive advantage in children should function as a "wake up call," borrowing from Dena Davis (Davis 1997), to prompt an ethical reflection on other problematic parental attitudes.

In this section I would like to challenge the arguments used to justify the use of genetic technologies to scout out children's athletic talents: is it always permissible or admirable for parents to "help" their children in such ways? It seems to me that the parental quality of nurturing children's talents is a degree-quality, i.e. it remains a quality only if exercised to a certain extent. If this is the case, it is legitimate to ask to what extent nurturing a talent is indeed an admirable attitude in parents, and above which, if any, threshold it ceases to be

---

6   A standardized test for most college admissions in the United States

admirable, and becomes actually of detriment to children. Therefore, instead of condoning new practices of talent-scouting and talent-nurturing on the basis of established old child-rearing practices, I think we should question the latter ones through the light shed by the former. Let us analyse a specific case: genetic tests to measure children's musical potential.

John Robertson has discussed the case of parents using genetic tests and PGD to select children with "perfect pitch." It is known that the gene for the perfect pitch runs in an autosomal dominant pattern, even though it has not been identified yet. (Robertson 2003, 464–466) Robertson imagines a future in which the gene has been identified, and where parents who have a strong interest in the musical abilities of their children may be willing to undergo IVF and PGD "to ensure this foundation for musical ability in their child." (Robertson 2003, 465) While the case discussed by Robertson remains a thought-experiment, it is not so far-fetched. The question is whether this request should be accepted or denied. Robertson argues that it should be accepted on the basis of the following argument: since parents "clearly have a right to instil or develop their child's musical ability after birth" (465) therefore, "they might plausibly argue that they should have that right before birth as well." But is this really the case? To what extent do parents have a right to instil and develop their children's musical ability? Do they have a right to do so from the age of 3, 4, or 5 years old? As a matter of fact, putting talented children in music or sports programs at the earliest possible age is necessary to maximize the particular option to become a successful professional in that field. But, if that is the case, how many hours a day, or a week, do parents have a right to impose musical exercises on their children? Do they have a right to do so at the expenses of children being "children," (i.e., experiencing childhood) on the basis that the goal of creating successful musicians justifies any means?

As mentioned above, Robertson justifies the use of genetic technologies to select children with the perfect pitch on the basis of older and more established practices of "nurturing" children's athletic talents, or of imposing on children the parental religion. Writes Robertson: "Parents … are free to instil and develop musical ability once the child is born, just as they are entitled to instil particular religious views." (Robertson 2003, 465) Contrary to Robertson, I do not think that the broad leeway parents currently have of inculcating their children with their religious views should be justified. Children should be left free to have a certain degrees of options open in front of them, so that they may flourish as full and autonomous human beings. Children should not be left to become the objects of parental aspirations and to fulfill their parents' expectation. It is important to reiterate that Robertson's example of the "perfect pitch" should not be considered only as a far-fetched thought experiment. As a matter of fact, parents are now able to resort to genetic tests sold online to scout out their children's potential for athletic performance, as I will detail in the next paragraph, and genetic tests to select for the perfect pitch may soon become available too.[7]

3.4 Direct-to-consumer genetic tests to "measure" athletic potential

As pointed out by Suter (2007), genetic technologies are particularly worrisome, as they open up a plethora of new ways in which parents can shape their children's ways and lives from very early on. In this section I analise the ethical implications of the recent boom of DTC genetic tests to – supposedly - measure children's athletic potential (Macur 2008; Stein 2011). This market is predominantly based in the United Stated, but not limited to it, as noted below.

In the United States, there are at least seven companies that sell DTC-genetic tests for sports performance or related traits. (Roth 2012) As the companies' data is proprietary, it is not clear exactly how many parents – and coaches! – are using these tests. A reasonable extrapolation puts the count in the order of several hundreds. (Brooks and Tarini 2011) In addition, since these tests are available on the Internet and quite affordable (in the range of $100-300), the market is not limited only to the US, but is open to potential customers in the UK, Europe or the rest of the world. Customers outside the US can order the test online and only have to pay higher shipping expenses for the test kit. It needs to be noted here that European regulations recommend, but do not

---

7   The following section first appeared in a slightly modified form in
     Sport, Ethics & Philosophy (2013): 7(2):175-185, title "Bend it like Beckham! The ethics of genetically testing children for athletic potential", doi :10.1080/17511321.2013.780183

require, genetic tests to be performed with a genetic counselling service. (Mc-Namee et al. 2009; Camporesi and McNamee 2013) With these tests, parents aim to gain an early advantage for their children, which would allow their children to turn already at an early age into professional athletes. In doing so, parents aim for an enhancement, which is seen mainly as a positional advantage.

What, if anything, is problematic with these practices? In the previous chapter I argued that parents should not be allowed to resort to PGD to choose to have deaf children like themselves, on the basis of the rights of the children to a/an (sufficiently) open future, and on the limits of parental reproductive freedom when it infringes on the children's capacity for self-determination. (Camporesi 2010) Compared to the use of PGD to conceive deaf children, the use of genetic technologies to scout out children's precocious athletic talents would seem *prima facie* to be a much less "radical" intervention, and as such it could be too easily dismissed as within the remit of parental education strategies. I would like to avoid here, though, such an easy dismissal.

To start with, it should be noted that the use of DTC- genetic tests does not always go alone, but at times can be paired to more 'traditional" methods for talent scouting, as a story published by the CNN shows. (Chang 2009) The story tells of a camp set up in Chongqing, a major city in south-west China. In the so-called "Children's Palace," about thirty children between the ages of 3 and 12 years old were selected to participate in an "innovative programme" that combined traditional methods of talent scouting with genetic testing, with the goal of providing Chinese children with "an effective, scientific plan [of development] at an early age" as put by Director Zhao Mingyou. (Chang 2009) The Chinese Government would then take care of implementing this "effective, scientific plan," by rearing the children in highly specialized academies or "boarding schools." An article appearing in the British tabloid Daily Mail during the London 2012 Olympics referred to these boarding schools as "talent factories", and pointed out that: "The school system causes family separation for weeks on end but the parents do not always mind. The socio-economic climate means many of them welcome the education their children receive. It is free, as are meals and accommodation." (McEvoy, 2012) While the example of a Chinese talent-scouting camp may seem far-fetched, cases of children reared in highly specialized academies are not inrefquent in the Western world, as the example of tennis champion Andre Agassi cited below demonstrates.

Most DTC-companies test for a panel of what they call "performance enhancing polymorphisms" (PEP). All of them test for the alpha-actinin 3 (ACTN3) polymorphism, which was the first PEP to be demonstrated to have an association with skeleto-muscle formation and function, and that I will describe in detail below. Although many genes and gene sequence variants have been tentatively associated with performance-related traits, few if any have risen to a level that would be called conclusive. As Roth (2012) recently pointed out: "This is not a judgment against the existing science, but rather a cognition of the infancy of the field of exercise and sports performance genomics." Not only is the field of genetics of sports performance in its infancy, but the DTC genetic tests use data obtained in one pool of subjects (i.e. elite athletes) and apply them to a substantially different one (i.e. children, teenagers) incurring the problem of "externality." (Eynon et al. 2011) As an example of this problem, I will focus on the test for ACTN3 polymorphism, which has the most robust scientific basis among the tests offered by the DTC companies. As mentioned above, ACTN3 was the first PEP to be demonstrated to have an association with skeleto-muscle formation and function, and is offered by all the companies available on the market. Therefore, any criticisms directed against this test will be valid also – and even more so – against the other tests, which rely on a shakier scientific basis.

In 2003, Yang et al. found a significantly higher frequency of the functional 477R genotype in the ACTN3 gene (where R stands in place of an arginine "R" rather than a stop codon) in both male and female elite sprinters. (Yang et al. 2003) Alfa-actinin is an actin-binding protein, where actin is an integral component of the protein superstructure that generates contractile force within muscle fibers. Polymorphisms in ACTN3 are thought to contribute to the heritability of fiber-type distribution in muscle, where the Type I are slow-twitch fibres that metabolise aerobically and are used in endurance races, while Type II are fast-twitch fibres that metabolise anaerobically, and are used in sprints. (Ostrander, Huson, and Ostrander 2009) The test for "ACTN3 Sports Gene" is sold as a genetic "Power/Speed performance test," and as we can read on the website of Atlas Sports Genetics[8] (one of the companies that

---

8   http://www.atlasgene.com/ [accessed March 18, 2014]

offer the test) with the aim to give "parents and coaches early information on their child's genetic predisposition for success in team or individual speed/ power or endurance sports." We can also read that the results of the tests will be "valuable in outlining training and conditioning programs necessary for athletic and sport development." (ibid.) The patent exploitation of the infancy of this field of research by the companies has been referred to by Caulfield (2011) as "scienceploitation," or the "exploitation of legitimate fields of science and, too often, patients and the general public, for profit and personal gain." A case in point for scienceploitation: the tests for ACTN3 variant claim to assess the predisposition to athletic ability and prowess, while the ACTN3 gene accounts for only 2% of total variance in muscle performance. (Eynon et al. 2011)

The rest of the variation is determined by a wide range of genetic and environmental factors, most of which (particularly the genetic factors) are very poorly understood. In addition, as pointed out by MacArthur (2008) (note that MacArthur is one of the authors who demonstrated the higher frequency of the ACTN3 polymorphism in elite sprinters), the fact that there is a higher frequency of ACTN3 polymorphism in elite sprinters does not mean that the test is actually predictive of athletic performance, (MacArthur 2008) as muscle performance (of which the ACTN3 variation accounts for only 2%) clearly does not equate with athletic prowess, notwithstanding what the companies are claiming. Finally, these tests pose a potential problem with false negatives, as the parents will act upon the results of these tests and the claims made by the companies and actively discourage their children from a particular kind of sports for which they allegedly do not have a genetic predisposition. For example, the company Geneffect frames the results of the ACTN3 test in terms of "genetic advantage" for "Sprint, Power & Strength Sports" for a RR genotype, for "Endurance Sports" for a XX genotype and for a "Mixed Pattern Sports" (equivalent for "any other sport") for a heterozygous genotype.[9]

Following a classification by Caulfield (2011) of DTC genetic tests into the three partially overlapping categories of: (a) the clearly preposterous; (b) the marginally pertinent; and (c) the vaguely predictive, we could say that, in a charitable interpretation, DTC genetic tests offered by companies such

---

9   http://www.geneffect.com/actn3/en/results.html [Accessed July 18, 2014]

as Atlas Sports Genetics, Sports X Factor, or Geneffect would be classified as marginally pertinent, while in a less charitable interpretation, they could be classified as clearly preposterous. Note that I am not saying here that the inability of DTC genetic tests to predict children's athletic performance is a matter of contingency in science or the infancy of the field. I think that DTC genetic tests will never be able to predict something as complex as athletic talent, even if the association were replicated in larger population samples and, therefore, strengthened. I am not interested in discussing the ethical implications of "GATTACA-like" science fiction scenarios where genetic tests are able to predict intelligence or other complex character traits as I agree wtih Atry and co-authors (2011) that it is the responsibility of the bioethicists not to create unwarranted hype concerning biomedical advancements. Athletic excellence is simply too complex a trait to be possibly pinned down to single or even multiple genetic associations in a deterministic fashion. This said, it is a matter of fact that information framed in terms of genetic knowledge appears to the public to be charged with an extra "authoritative aura" that seems to be intrinsic in the G, A, T and C bases of the deoxyribonucleic acid. It is also a matter of fact that these companies market their tests, and that at least some parents accept their results, as if they were deterministic in nature, and as if they were really able to predict the talent of their children. Therefore, parents act upon these tests and make decisions on the basis of the results that involve investing in their children's future. By doing so, the tests acquire a causal significance in the lives of these children. In what follows I will analyse the ethical permissibility of the parental practices independent of the above criticism on the scientific validity of the claim.

Brad Marston, father of nine-year-old prospective soccer player Elizabeth, is a satisfied customer and a testimonial for Atlas Sport Genetics. His testimonial can be read on the company website:[10]

> Atlas Sports Genetics testing was very informative and the process was quite simple. Although my daughter is only 9 she now knows that she has the "Sprint, Power, & Strength advantage" which we can use to market her athletic career and hopefully a wonderful scholarship from this process.

---

10   http://www.atlasgene.com/index.php?do=testimonial [Accessed July 18, 2014]

As already mentioned above, Brad Marston does not represent the emergence of a new kind of parent. On the contrary, he represents a new instance of parents who employ all available methods to steer their children towards a life of athletic, musical or other early professionalism. Parents have always done so: from submitting their children to heavy training schedules, to intensive summer camps, to hiring private teachers and tutors, and so on and so forth. These kinds of attitudes can be reinforced by the consequences, i.e. if the child becomes a successful professional in her field, her success seems to confirm the "rightness" of the childrearing parental behaviour, in a kind of retroactive approval that takes the form of: "See, it was worth it" or "I was right in the end," etc. DTC genetic tests aimed at measuring the athletic potential of a child can be seen as the latest tool available to parents to steer their children's future, and their investments, with the expectation that their efforts will be – quite literally – "paid off." Is it justifiable for parents to do so?

Feinberg has defined the child's right to an open future (ROF) as a "vague formula that describes the form of the particular rights in question but not their content."(Feinberg 1980a) The rights in question are "rights in trust," or anticipatory autonomy rights: they look like adult autonomy rights, except that the child cannot exercise her choice until later on in life. The violation means that when the child is an autonomous adult, certain key options will be already closed to her, undermining her capacity for self-determination (which Feinberg sees as a necessary condition for self-fulfillment in life). As already noted by Dixon (2007), Mills objects to Feinberg and argues that not only is it impossible to actually have an open future due to the finitude of our lives, and to the inevitable closure of possibilities that takes place every time we make a choice, but also that it would not even be a desirable option. (Mills 2003) For Mills, parental approaches that aim to leave their children with an open future consequently expose them to a frenetic "smorgasbord" of activities, and end up being detrimental to a vision of more profound and authentic experiences of the life of a child. This more profound vision would encompass also a meaningful "idleness," a time for play that is not necessarily goal-directed (to success, or fame), and that privileges the child *hic et nunc* vs. the successful and possibly burnt-out adult that the child will grow into.

I find the analysis by Mills very compelling: it seems true to me that some parents are constantly projecting into the future of their children, and do not give a proper value to the present child that they have in front of them. What was once "free time" from school and homework has become time devoted to activities x, y, z, which by virtue of being activities that are goal-directed (talent-scout, talent-development directed) lose their value of free, idle time that is supposed to act as a counterbalance to the already many compulsory activities that a child has to undertake early on in life. But, as Mianna Lotz has correctly pointed out, this is only half the story. (Lotz 2006) Lotz, while recognizing the validity of some of the worries raised by Mills against the smorgasbord approach adopted by some parents, shows that such criticisms are not really directed to Feinberg's, but to current trends of childrearing and educating driven by excessively competitive parents. In other words, striving to protect a child's ROF does not commit parents to the problematic "smorgasbord attitudes" described by Mills. Indeed, if we look back at the original source, we can see that Feinberg is well aware of the inevitable narrowing of options in parenting:

> Simply by living their own lives as they choose, the parents will be forming an environment around the child that will tend to shape his budding loyalties and habits. (Feinberg 1980, 735)

This narrowing of possible futures is inevitable in the practice of parenting and especially so in the case of talented children, but does not necessarily violate the child's ROF, provided that the child's input is taken, whenever possible, into consideration. How is that possible in practice?

David Archard also argues along similar lines that parents cannot avoid (nor would it be desirable if they tried) forming their children's characters to some extent. He writes: "It would be a caricature of ideal liberal parents to imagine them zealously striving to avoid the creation of any particular personality in their children." (Archard 2004, 56-7) Archard acknowledges that the choices made by parents concerning their children's rearing and education have an "opportunity" cost for their children, namely the absence of some other upbringing, but this is unavoidable. Moreover, self-determination of the child is not the only value to take into account when evaluating upbringing. A good upbringing should realize the child's talents, and these may be realized sometimes only to the detriment of self-determination, and, therefore, of the child's open future. Talented children are particularly difficult cases, as the nurturing of a precocious musical or sport talent may lead to a successful adult (concert soloist, Wimbledon tennis player, etc.), but that will have been achieved at the expenses of other skills (possibly, all other skills except that particular one which was nurtured) and of the person's self-determination. How is it then possible to preserve the child's budding sense of self-determination, while also nurturing her talents? As said above, Feinberg's analysis of the children's ROF is that of a "right in trust," i.e. a right to be saved for the child until she becomes an adult. I will now try to combine Feinberg's ROF with an analysis of what it means for a child to become an adult, and what implications this process has on the development of the child's autonomy.

Tamar Schapiro addresses a very important but fairly neglected question: what is a child, such that it could be appropriate to treat a person like one? (Schapiro 1999) In tackling this question, Schapiro is addressing also the following two related questions: (a) When is a parent justified in preventing a child from acting according to her own will? and (b) When is a child entitled to make her own choices? Schapiro draws a parallel between children being provisional, passive members of the political community and children also being provisional, passive members of the ethical community. Their status of passivity is provisional because of their liminal and ever-changing status, and their condition of moving towards adulthood. Indeed, as children at different stages of development differ from one another in the extent to which they have hegemony over themselves, they also differ in the relative status of their passivity as members of the ethical community. Children gain access to the ethical community once they gain autonomy and sovereignty, as put by Schapiro, by developing increasingly broader "domains of discretion." Once they have achieved sovereignty over some domain of discretion (e.g. being able to eat without being fed, being able to get dressed alone, being able to choose which clothes to wear, and so on and so forth), children should be left to decide and exercise autonomy over that domain. In this way, writes Schapiro, the child is forced to come up with provisional principles of deliberation that function then as starting points, as anchors, for "ever widening domains of discretion." Along similar lines, Feinberg writes: "The child can [and should, I would add] contribute towards the making of his own self and circumstances in ever-increasing degree." (Feinberg 1980b, 736) This contribution to her own self-determination entails, I think, also exercising her autonomy over the sport she (the child) wants to play, or does not want to play. Parental attitudes exemplified by the use of DTC genetic tests to provide children with a "head start" in life are deeply problematic because – as put by Wall (2010) – they interpret children "only through the lens of what they are not yet, namely adults" (Wall 2010, 144) and do not take into account the *in fieri* moral agency of the child. Borrowing again from Wall, while at first glance it may seem an obvious goal that the main purpose of parenting is "helping children to grow up into adults," this practice "obscures the ethical sense in which children are diverse and other moral agents in and of themselves." (Wall 2010, 144) Children should expect from their parents to be equipped with a range of broad skills that will enable them to make autonomous decisions and choose their path in life. On the converse, being equipped with very specific skills (like playing pre-professionally soccer, football, volleyball and so on) very early in life and having a life plan spelled out for them would constitute a brake on their development, and relegate them to being passive receivers of education. In addition, by depriving children of the possibility to exercise their budding self-determination, it relegates them to being passive members of the moral community. The possession of a "life plan" early on in life has been defined by Slote as both "unnatural" and "unfortunate." (Slote 1989, 40–41) "Life-planfulness" as a character-trait is seen by Slote as a virtue with a temporal aspect, i.e. a "positively good thing in individuals mature enough ... to decide upon a career or profession," but a trait that can become an obstacle for development in children, a "brake" to the existence itself of their autonomic domains of discretion.

Returning to the focus of our analysis: What about children with talents? Slote recognizes that an early start can be necessary for the fulfillment of that talent, as he writes:

> All this [considering a life plan a bad thing in children] is consistent with allowing that those who make premature life plans concerning careers are sometimes very successful in those careers. But such premature choices are typically the result of parental pressure, and those who yield to, and succeed under, such pressure can hardly help being emotionally scarred by it as well. (Slote 1989, 47)

Talented children are, indeed, particularly challenging for educators, as the nurturing of a precocious musical or sport talent is often essential to the realization a successful adult. The examples of successful adults (musicians, athletes, mathematicians, artists) who had a very difficult if not miserable childhood as talented kids or prodigies are abundant. (Solomon 2012) An example that comes to mind is Andre Agassi, the American Hall of Fame tennis player whose father allegedly tied a tennis racket to Andre's hand when he was only three years old, and obliged him to hit tennis ball after tennis ball that were being literally spit out by a dragon-like machine built specifically for that purpose. (Agassi 2010) In his autobiography, Andre Agassi is very resentful towards his father and the education he was submitted to: even though Andre grew up to be one of the world's most famous tennis players, he achieved that at the expenses of all other skills, including basic school education. Note also that both of Andre's older siblings, being also talented children in tennis, were submitted to a similar education, but never made it to a professional career. Not only does this constitute an ethical issue for the infringement of the child's capacity for self determination, but it is also an ethical issue for the infringement and the lack of capacity of understanding the person in front of us at that very moment, i.e. the child.

To reiterate this important point, talented children are tough cases exactly because they embody the tension between nurturing talent and the self-determination capacity of the child, both of which are considered duties of a good parent. Indeed, it can be plausible to argue that the particular kind of precocious and "absolutist" upbringing necessary to nurture the child's talent was the only possible way to achieve success in a domain where early training and gaining of a competitive advantage is essential. It seems, therefore, that parents must strive both to realize the child's particular talents and at the same time to safeguard her "open future." This is no easy task for parents trying to keep a difficult balance between the good of this particular child (realising the present) and the good of the adult that the child will grow up to be (the future). The tension between these two goals will be exacerbated when these goals are defined in maximizing terms, i.e. the Andre Agassi or the concert soloist at Royal Albert Hall.

As noted by Mike McNamee and co-authors, if it is appropriate to characterize the field of "sports ethics" as in its infancy, then it is even more appropriate to characterize the field of "sports medicine ethics" as neonatal. (McNamee et al. 2009) The analysis of genetic tests for athletic performance falls within this "neonatal" realm. Note also that the comment by Roth (2012) on the infancy of exercise and sports genomics falls along similar lines. Both (elite) sports and medicine can be defined as goal-directed activities: the former as having "victory" as one of its goals, the latter "health." Both "victory" and "health" are regarded as goods by the subjects involved in the activities, and these goals may very well be, and often are, in contrast in elite sports (think for example of return to play decisions after injury). (Mathias 2004) As noted by Mathias, "The history of ethics in sports medicine has been driven by the general tension between the demands of sport and the demands of health" (Mathias 2004, 196) and, therefore, we should "not be surprised to find in the field where they come together, sports medicine, signs of this tension occur in the form of persistent ethical problems" (ibid.). The aim of sports in children, though, need not necessarily be "victory." Quite on the contrary, I think that sport in children should not be a goal-directed activity (directed to victory), differently from what it is for the athlete who is engaged in a professional, elite sport. Sport in children could instead be understood as a "practice," defined by MacIntyre as a coherent and complex form of socially established cooperative human activity, through which goods internal to that form of activity are realized in the course of trying to achieve those standards of excellence which are appropriate to, and partially definitive of, that form of activity. (MacIntyre 1984, 186) In this sense, sport as a practice in childhood becomes defined both by goods internal to the practice (e.g. to stay healthy, enjoy the company of friends, enjoy the discovery of the possibilities of one's own body, learn how to relate with a team, learn the importance of rules, etc.) and by the standards of excellence of the practice (i .e. nurturing and developing talent). Returning to Slote and his analysis of the temporality of virtues, we could also add that some goods are intrinsic to childhood (including engaging in a sport as a practice, and not as in a competitive profession directed to victory) and as such should be preserved. Therefore, parents could, and should, expose children to a variety of sport activities (and other non sport-related activities) compatible with their financial situations, and their own preferences and ways of living. In this sense, I think that parents could and indeed should be free to live "their own lives as they choose," as put by Feinberg (quoted above), as long as they "do not isolate children intentionally from other ways of life, and make sure that children learn of the variety of ways of life." (Lotz 2006, 541)

To conclude, I recognize the existence of an unavoidable tension between the goal of maximizing children's talents and nurturing their self-determination, but I am inclined to view the latter as more important. Nonetheless, I recognize the impossibility and non-desirability of non-directiveness in childrearing, and I find the criticism by Mills of "smorgasbord" parental attitudes quite appropriate and resonant with current Western trends of parenting. These arguments form my two-pronged rationale to object to the parental use of DTC genetic tests to (supposedly) measure their children's athletic potential, and to steer their education towards an early start to a professional sports career. In the next section I move on to considering anti-doping governance, and I analyse the arguments in favour of allowing doping under a medical context.

3.5 Performance enhancement and anti-doping governance: towards doping under medical context?

As illustrated already earlier on in this chapter, professional sport has always been a laboratory for biomedical and biotechnological innovations regarding the treatment of injury, recovery and training regimes aimed at maximising athletic performance. It is a matter of fact that elite athletes are willing to accept high degrees of risks in exchange for the expected performance enhancing benefits derived from the consumption of substances, from extreme training regimes or diets, to the experimentation upon themselves of innovative surgeries. It is also a matter of fact that athletes often lack information on the safety and effectiveness of the agents they are taking, or of the performance enhancing technologies that they are undertaking.

This happens because the existing WADA Code (now subject to revisions expected to come into effect in January 2015) does not require that a substance has a demonstrably performance enhancing effect for it to be included on the Prohibited List. At present, it suffices that the substance has the "potential" to enhance athletic performance, in addition to meeting one of the other two criteria of the definition of doping already illustrated in section 3.1: that it is harmful (or potentially so), or that it is against the spirit of sport. (WADA

Code 2012) Therefore, the lack of information on the safety and effectiveness of the performance enhancing agents that are introduced in the practice of professional sport means that in some cases athletes may be actually taking on the risks of the drugs, without experiencing any performance enhancing effect. In addition, the athletes lack protection against the conflict of interest that can arise in the professional sport context, where short-term gains (such as a swifter return to play after an injury) and the gaining of "competitive edge" are often in conflict with the long-term health of the athlete-subject. (Huizenga 1995; Nixon 1993; Howe 2004)

King and Robeson note how well understood problems in research ethics (i.e., vulnerability, voluntariness, undue influence, full disclosure, equitable subject selections, conflict of interest) become particularly problematic in the elite sports context, as opposed to the more typical health, medical and scientific contexts in and through which research is already regulated. (King and Robeson 2007) To the best of my knowledge, King and Robeson were the first authors to bring to the fore the problematic position of the athlete-patient, situated in a professional sport context where the introduction of performance enhancing technologies can be regarded as "unregulated clinical research." (King and Robeson 2007) King and Robeson also note how, in the current system where performance enhancing substances and technologies are introduced into athletes' bodies, which become the locus of unregulated experimentation, three types of potentially serious consequences follow:

> First, the people who receive the innovation lack information about it, particularly about the limits of knowledge about it. Second, they lack protection against the conflicts of interest that can arise when the innovator has more than the individual's well-being in mind (such as product development). Finally, the safety and effectiveness of the innovation cannot be adequately determined. (King and Robeson 2007, 5-6)

Finally, they define athletes as "unwitting or unwilling research subjects," or "guinea pigs." As mentioned above, the WADC is currently under revision, and it appears that the 2015 Code will elevate "performance enhancement" from being merely one of three criteria to a necessary condition of doping, to be supported by either of both of the remaining (now) secondary conditions: harm to health and contrariness to the spirit of sport. (McNamee 2012) Nevertheless, as I argue extensively in my co-authored paper (Camporesi and McNamee 2014), if the performance enhancing criterion indeed becomes a necessary condition, there should be reasonable grounds for a product's or process' inclusion on the Prohibited List – reasonable grounds that, at the moment, do not appear to be evident, as many of the substances included in the Prohibited List are merely presumed to be ergogenic. Therefore, in (Camporesi and McNamee 2014), we argue that a proper governance framework would need to be established both to assess the performance enhancing effects of the substances, and the risks to the health of the athlete. I am aware that sometimes it will be inevitable that the inclusion of a substance on the Prohibited List will involve reasonable extrapolation. For instance, there is good evidence to suggest that the use of beta-blockers enhances performance in pistol shooting (Kruse et al. 1986; Silver 2001) and that this might be contrary to the spirit of sport, as it infringes the level-playing field which is a necessary condition for fairness equality in competition. (Camporesi and McNamee 2014) Thus beta-blockers are reasonably banned and considered doping. Yet we dispute that the ban applies not only to target sports – where the inference is reasonable – but also to other sports, where its performance enhancing effects seem less than obvious. To be clear, we would not count as reasonable grounds anecdotal evidence on performance enhancing effects or harmful effects of a substance, such as creatine with (say) a particular population (children). (Calfee and Fadale 2006)

As shown in section 3.1, the negative connotation of doping practices is a relatively recent acquisition. More recently, there has been a return to those initial arguments, and several authors have argued in favour of legalising doping. For one, see Foddy, Savulescu and Clayton, who argue that doping is not contrary to the spirit of sport (Savulescu, Foddy, and Clayton 2004), or Andy Miah, who argues that a pro-doping culture will not only be inevitable in the future of professional sports, but that it is also an essential part of what we value in sport (and of why we are interested in it), i.e., pushing humanity to its limits and beyond. (Miah 2006) Atry and co-authors have argued in favour of establishing a shared responsibility for doping, which is not limited to the athletes, but would include also the sponsors, the fans, and in general all the relevant stakeholders in elite sports. (Atry et al. 2012; Atry 2013)

In the next chapter I continue this discussion and consider the charge that such arguments could lead to doping under a medical context, by analysing the perspective put forward by Holm (2007), and providing a possible alternative to alter the payoff matrix in professional sport, without allowing doping under a medical context. I will also discuss the place of enhancement research in society, and attempt to lay the ground for shifting the discussion of enhancements from the ethical to the political level.

Chapter 4

Shifting the debate on enhancements from the ethical to the political level

4.1 A proposal to alter the payoff matrix in professional sports: shifting the burden of proof of doping to sponsors

It is a matter of fact that professional athletes often discount their future health in exchange for desired enhanced performances.[1] Some recent examples include Kobe Bryant of the Los Angeles Lakers, who publicly challenged teammate Dwight Howard to play through a torn labrum in his shoulder: "We don't have time for [Howard's shoulder] to heal," said Bryant (MacMullan 2013). In another example from the United States, National Football League athletes continue to play through concussions and head trauma, leading to long-term brain damage that has been linked to chronic traumatic encephalopathy (permanent brain damage associated with early-onset dementia), with disastrous consequences for the life of the footballer after his career. (Schwarz 2009; Kotz 2012) Professional athletes also discount their future health by engaging in doping behaviours. Commenting upon the recent doping scandals of Jamaican track & field athletes (Asafa Powell, Sherone Simson and three other world-class sprinters tested positive for the banned substance Oxylofrine in the summer of 2013), Dr Paul Wright, a senior drug tester with the Jamaican Anti-Doping Commission (JADCO), said in an interview to the BBC that the

---

1   This section and the next one first appeared in a longer version for
    Reflective Practice 2014, volume 15, issue 1, co-authored with James A.
    Knuckles with title "Shifting the burden of proof in doping: lessons from
    environmental sustainability applied to highperformance sport" and doi:
    10.1080/14623943.2013.86920

scandals represented only "the tip of the iceberg." (Bond 2013) Wright added that since these tests occurred in competition, the athletes knew "months before" when and where they would be tested, leading Wright to infer that many more athletes must be planning their doping around competitions so as not to get caught. (Bond 2013)

Cases like these abound because high-performance athletes are focused more on their athletic achievements now than their future health status. They adopt therefore a "win at all costs attitude" as described by Krumer and co-authors (2011) that discounts future health for current athletic success. This becomes the middle step in a three-rung ladder towards doping, where money from sponsors based on records, recognition, and victories, leads to a win-at-all-cost mentality, which in turn leads to strong incentives for athletes to dope. Therefore, a vicious link between money and doping aimed at a constant improvement of performances takes place, with the consequence that professional sport may not be sustainable as a practice, both because athletes harm themselves by engaging in doping practices, and because uncoupling money from increased competition and quest for records and recognition is unlikely to happen under the current system.

How to alter this "discounting"? One solution might be to lift the ban on doping, and redefine it in a medical context. Indeed, this solution was recently presented by several authors, including Miah (2006), Savulescu, Foddy and Clayton (2004), and Savulescu (2013). As shown by Holm (2007) though (see discussion below), even if the ban on doping were to be lifted and doping were to be placed under "medical control," athletes would still have incentives to dope clandestinely, and a two-tiered system of doping would ensue. How to escape this seeming "Catch-22"? Here we propose an alternative way to alter the practice of high-performance athletes discounting their future health for current performance, without engaging in doping under a medical context, by shifting the burden of proof from the regulator and athlete to the private sector (i.e. sponsors), as well as providing the right incentives in the form of penalties to the sponsors for athletes found positive. In order to do so, we learn from similar discussions in the sustainability field, where it has long been proposed to shift the burden of proof of damaging the environment from regulators to the private sector.

Altering the discounting of the future health of professional athletes

Krumer et al. (2011) conducted a survey among professional athletes to measure subjective time discounting. Their sample included 74 professional Israeli athletes from different sports and 70 non-athletes in the control. The survey asked participants to indicate how much they would be willing to pay now in order to postpone a future payment (e.g., pay $10 now to postpone a $20 debt), and how much they would be willing to receive now in lieu of receiving a payment in the future (e.g., receive $10 now instead of $15 next month) (Krumer, Shavit, and Rosenboim 2011). As expected, the results suggested that "athletes discounted time more heavily than non-athletes" (i.e., the athletes more strongly preferred access to money in the present than non-athletes). The authors argue convincingly that athletes' time preference is affected by their sport orientation and a "win at all costs attitude." Waldron and Krane (2005) have also described the adoption of what they refer to as "whatever it takes" attitude in female professional athletes, who increasingly engage in health compromising behaviours such as playing when injured, sacrificing their bodies, and overtraining. Waldron and Krane write that "while the mind focuses on winning at any costs, the body can be compromised for the good of the cause" (Waldron and Krane 2005, 320), and describe how athletes endorse hiding pain and injury through an attitude of "irreverence" which can be, and very often is, very detrimental to the future health of the athlete.

Gymnastics offers one famous example: Kerri Strug, the US gymnast who vaulted through a sprained ankle to ensure the US gold medal in the 1996 Olympics. (Weinberg 2004) While her desire to push her body beyond its limits was not likely a result of her hoping it would land her a large endorsement contract, the sponsor endorsements that followed as a result of her bravery (in fact, after the 1996 Olympics, General Mills corporation featured her on the front of the Wheaties cereal box, and Strug received additional sponsorship from Visa corporation and others) did send a strong message to other athletes: if you push through pain, and become a hero, you will win a large sponsorship contract. An article written in the Chicago Tribune in 1996 aptly captured this sentiment:

Even Nike, the quasi-spiritual sportswear monster, praises pain in a commercial that flashes images of boxers with bloodied faces, runners falling
and grimacing, and some sorry competitor vomiting. Just do it. No pain, no
gain. Whatever it takes. What does not kill me makes me stronger. (Gregory
1996)

Gymnastics may in fact be one of the sports where the win-at-all-costs attitude is most widespread in very young female athletes, who are often subjected to tortuous professional-style training when they are toddlers (Cintado
2007; Giordano 2010). In China, for example, Nanning Gymnasium Camp
was recently featured by the UK Daily Mail magazine which portrayed har-
rowing pictures of toddlers crying for pain while being subjected to strenu-
ous sessions that border on psychological and physical torture. (Blake 2012)
Nanning Camp is not an isolated example but one of many training camps
where children no older than 5 or 6 years old are sent by their parents to "learn
to become champions" from an early age in preparation for the Olympics.
(Blake 2012) More recently, these camps have been coupled to genetic tests
to scout out children's talents, as described in the previous chapter. These
examples clearly illustrate instances of professional athletes sacrificing tomor-
row's health for today's victory.

As a result of this win-at-all-costs mentality, many athletes turn to doping
to gain a competitive edge in their sport. One solution that has been proposed
in this context might be to lift the ban on doping. For one example, see Foddy,
Savulescu and Clayton, who argue that doping is not contrary to the spirit of
sport, (Savulescu, Foddy, and Clayton 2004; Savulescu 2013) or Andy Miah,
who argues that a pro-doping culture will not only be inevitable in the future
of increasingly technological sports at the elite level, but that it is also an essential part of what we value in sport (and of why we are interested in it),
i.e., pushing humanity to its limits and beyond. (Miah 2006) Commenting in
the press on the recent doping scandals of American sprinter Tyson Gay and
Jamaican sprinters Asafa Powell and Sherone Simpson, Savulescu has argued
that:

To keep improving, to keep beating records, to continue to train at the peak
of fitness, to recover from the injury that training inflicts, we need enhanced

physiology. Spectators want faster times and broken records, so do athletes. But we have exhausted the human potential. Is it wrong to aim for zero tolerance and performances that are within natural human limits? No, but it is not enforceable (Savulescu 2013)

Savulescu therefore proposes to legalise doping, or to put doping "under medical control." This type of solution has been addressed and refuted by Holm (2007). Holm spells out the two possible scenarios that would take place were a ban on doping to be lifted. In the first scenario, athletes have access to data on the effectiveness and side effects of the performance enhancing substances; while in the second scenario athletes get impartial advice from the sports doctor about when and how to dope. (Holm 2007) Importantly, Holm argues that in both scenarios, athletes would still have incentives to cheat, and a two-tiered system of doping (under a medical context and of secretive doping) would ensue. Athletes have strong incentives to keep doping practices secretive in order to maintain an exclusive use on a drug, and therefore a competitive advantage over fellow athletes. Holm identifies these incentives as an instance of a "take and hide" option that dominates other options in a Prisoner's Dilemma-style coordination game, the other options being not doping or doping and being open about it. In addition, as Holm points out, more often than not, the athlete's income is controlled by his/her employer (e.g. team and, ultimately, sponsor), and the degree of control that the athlete has over the decision to play/to compete is often limited. For these reasons, Holm describes how it is not lifting the ban on doping that will incentivize athletes to stop doping, but changing the "payoff matrix," characterised by high financial rewards for current athletic success. (Holm 2007, 139) In the next section we describe tools from the sustainability field that could be very useful when applied to the field of professional sport to change the payoff matrix, and therefore to alter the practice of athletes discounting their future health.

4.2 What can high-performance sports learn from the field of environmental sustainability?

In the sustainability field, we can draw parallels to each of the three elements of our argument outlined above: setting the principle, levying penalties, and enforcing the regulations. Regarding the first element, it has long been argued that the burden of proof in cases of damages to the environment should not be on the relevant regulatory agency or local community, but instead should be on the entities whose actions might cause environmental damage. This concept of shifting the burden of proof has its roots in Principle 15 of the Rio Declaration, set forth at the United Nations Conference on Environment and Development in Rio de Janeiro, Brazil, in 1992. (United Nations 1992) Often referred to as the Precautionary Principle, it was first proposed as:

> In order to protect the environment, the precautionary approach shall be widely applied by States according to their capabilities. Where there are threats of serious or irreversible damage, lack of full scientific certainty shall not be used as a reason for postponing cost-effective measures to prevent environmental degradation. (UN 1992)

More recent forms of the precautionary principle now often include a statement on burden of proof. This addition was brought to the forefront of international sustainability governance in 1997 with a high-level workshop in Lisbon, Portugal commissioned by the Independent World Commission on the Oceans and subsequent article in which the now famous principles for governing the world's oceans in a sustainable way was published. Known as the Lisbon Principles of Sustainable Governance, the third principle states:

> In the face of uncertainty about potentially irreversible environmental impacts, decisions concerning their use should err on the side of caution. *The burden of proof should shift to those whose activities potentially damage the environment.* [emphasis added] (Costanza et al. 1998)

The crux of this statement rests in its call for any entity whose actions could potentially damage the oceans to prove before and during the action that they are not doing any damage. Turning to the second element of our argument – penalties – we see that the Lisbon Principles do not mention penalties (or enforcement, which we address below). Yet other scholars have argued that the penalties for environmental damage should be proportional to the damages that are caused and should be imposed on the entity responsible for the damage. Segerson and Tietenberg (1992) analysed penalties for environmental infractions, and conclude first that fines are preferable to incarceration because "the social costs associated with incarceration are so much higher." (Segerson and Tietenberg 1992, 180) They then conclude that "a fine should be imposed on each party [that damages the environment] in an amount equal to the damages that result from its actions." (Segerson and Tietenberg 1992, 181) Finally, they find that fines should be levied against the organization and not the individual, primarily because events that lead to environmental damage are usually the result of a complex chain of actions and responsibilities within the organization (Segerson and Tietenberg 1992).

In practice, however, while penalties – and liability – might fall on the organization and generally favour financial penalties over incarceration, it is difficult if not impossible to set the penalty at a level equal to the costs of the damage. First, limits on total liability for a company enshrined in law can prevent regulatory agencies from seeking penalties that match the costs of the damages. For example, the Canadian government limits "absolute liability" for offshore oil and gas drilling companies to CA$ 1 billion (for comparison, 2010 estimates of the BP oil spill in the Gulf of Mexico put the cost at around US$ 40 billion). (Wearden 2010; Rozmus 2013) Second, it can be very difficult to calculate the total costs of a particular damaging event or action, particularly because calculating economic costs of environmental damage is difficult and imprecise. Using the BP oil spill as an example again, a panel of experts has recently concluded that the United States government, after extensive research and countless studies, has still failed to determine the true costs of the disaster because it incorrectly and incompletely accounted for the economic costs of the loss of environmental services as a result of the oil spill. (National Research Council 2013)

As to the question of enforcement – enforcing penalties, conducting testing and monitoring, and taking regulatory action – a recent example comes from the US chemical industry. In their 2009 paper, Schwarzman and Wilson state:

> Given the size of the chemical enterprise, the extent to which it is woven into the fabric of society, and the backlog of unexamined chemicals, a new approach is needed that does not rely on resource-intensive, chemical-bio-

> chemical risk assessments in which government, at great public expense,
> bears the burden of proof. (Wilson and Schwarzman 2009, 1202)

This "new approach" is characterized by requiring chemical companies to prove their chemicals are safe, rather than waiting for the regulator to test each chemical. Addressing the issue of enforcement, Wilson and Schwarzman (2009) argue that because the US regulator – in this case, the Environmental Protection Agency – currently bears the full burden of proving whether or not a chemical causes environmental (or health) harm, it must obtain a high-level of certainty that the chemical is causing harm before setting its machinations in motion to take regulatory action against the chemical company. Furthermore, the chemical companies keep secret as much information on their chemicals as possible, and are known to either withhold information or create misleading information, causing the regulatory agency to doubt whether it has sufficient grounds to take regulatory action. (Wilson and Schwarzman 2009) In industries like the chemical manufacturing industry, where the very activities that drive profit can cause environmental harm, only the private sector has the capacity, information, and resources necessary to conduct adequate testing required to prove that their actions are not causing environmental damage. Enforcement – and imposing fines for noncompliance – is still the responsibility of the regulator, however, and the regulator needs to maintain its own testing in order to fully enforce its policies and effectively shift the burden of proof onto the private sector.

After more than twenty years of discussions around shifting the burden of proof away from regulators, it seems therefore that the current system in the field of sustainability is advancing slowly towards a higher degree of accountability of the companies for the consequences of their actions on the environment. Still, in the majority of cases when a company damages the environment, the burden of proof remains on the damaged region/community and relevant regulator to show that it was the company's fault. The process has been especially slow in the oil and gas industry, whose normal business operations can result in environmental harm. Companies in this industry therefore will strongly resist efforts to require them to prove that their actions are not damaging the environment, and in most cases, it remains the responsibility of the local authorities and regulatory agency to detect and prove environmental damage.

In the examples above that describe shifting burdens of proof away from regulators and onto entities whose actions might damage the environment, we see that setting the general principle of identifying a level of penalty (e.g., equal to the damages that a chemical spill caused) is relatively straightforward. However, actually calculating that penalty (e.g., it may be easy to calculate the immediate clean up cost, but what about long-term effects like increased cancer risk or biodiversity loss?), or being legally allowed to impose the full amount, as well as enforcing regulations, has proven difficult in the sustainability field. As we will see below, these difficulties also carry over to the field of professional sports.

We can now draw some important lessons from the sustainability field and apply them to the professional sport context. First, the burden of proof principle can be translated to the sports context as the following: the burden of proof should shift to those whose activities may lead to doping in athletic competitions. We can also see that it is important to shift the burden of proof to the entities with the resources available to conduct case-by-case monitoring and testing (e.g., the chemical companies in the example above, and not the US EPA). Given these two lessons learned, and the link between sponsorship and doping that we highlight earlier, we argue that the burden of proof should be shifted to the companies that sponsor professional athletes. It should be the sponsors' responsibility to prove that each athlete they sponsor is "clean" before they sponsor him or her, and throughout the sponsorship contract.

Second, we see from the environmental sustainability examples that setting penalties on the organization and not the individual is preferable, as are financial penalties as opposed to incarceration. We argue similarly for the high-performance sports context: penalties should be imposed on the sponsoring organizations, and not on the specific individuals in the organizations responsible for the contract with the athlete who is found to be doping. The entity of the penalty should not be based on the costs of the damage caused by doping, but instead on amounts that would significantly impact the sponsoring company's financials (e.g., a percentage of the previous year's earnings), and without a maximum cap. Calculating a penalty based on publicly available financial data for the sponsoring companies is significantly easier (and less disputable) than calculating a penalty based on the social, economic, and health costs of doping.

Third, we argue for WADA's continued enforcement of its anti-doping policies, with strengthened testing capabilities and research into doping methods and technologies, in addition to what it already does.[2] Strengthening its testing and research capacity and capabilities is important because if WADA finds that an athlete has been doping, it levies the penalty on the sponsoring companies irrespective of any test results that the sponsoring companies provide to WADA. WADA's testing determines whether an athlete has been doping, not the sponsors' testing; therefore, WADA's tests set the *de facto* testing standard for the sponsorship companies. The sponsors will undoubtedly conduct their own testing to verify that their athletes are clean, but if a WADA-initiated test finds that an athlete has been doping, the WADA test overrides any tests that the sponsor conducted.

Conversely, in the current system in professional sport, when an athlete turns out positive for doping, the sponsors dump her/him (and often sue him/her), while all along they had been closing one or both eyes to the practice of doping because they had an interest in the athlete continuing to win. The athlete suffers tremendously – in both financial, social and potentially health-related costs – and the sport as a whole suffers a tarnished reputation. The sponsors' images may be similarly tarnished, but usually for a much briefer time period, and at a far lower cost relative to their overall financial position. Yet, it was the sponsors' collective money that essentially paid for the athlete's doping, and created a win-at-all-costs mentality in the sport. Recent examples include Lance Armstrong and professional cycling illustrated below, several prominent athletes in the US Major League Baseball Association, (McLean 2013) and Marion Jones as a Track & Field star. (CNN Associated Press 2007)

Let us take a closer look at Lance Armstrong's case, for example. Lance has been one of the most successful, if not the most successful, road cyclist in modern history, winning the Tour de France seven consecutive times between 1999 and 2005, achieving an all-time record which has now been revoked as he was disqualified and banned for life from competition by United States

---

2   The full list of up-to-date WADA-funded research projects can be found here: http://www.wada-ama.org/en/science-medicine/research/funded-research-projects/ [accessed July 18, 2014]

Anti-Doping Agency (USADA) in 2012. After years of denials and lawsuits against those who accused him of doping, Lance admitted publicly to doping in January 2013, in an interview on television conducted by Oprah Winfrey (Winfrey 2013). The now "disgraced" Lance Armstrong faces a plethora of lawsuits: the Sunday Times, which Armstrong had previously sued in 2006 for alleging he was doping (The Guardian Associated Press 2013); the US Justice Department for the US$ 40 million that the US Postal Service spent to sponsor Lance's cycling team from 1998 to 2004 (Frieden 2013); and a group of discontented readers in California for false memoirs which were sold as non-fiction (yes, that is true). (Bury 2013) While we will not comment on the other lawsuits here as they fall outside the direct scope of this paper, we would contend that it seems unlikely that the US Postal Service was completely unaware of Armstrong's doping, or at least they remained purposefully unaware by not conducting their own testing. In this way, one could argue that the USPS was in some ways complicit in the doping activities (and indeed benefited financially from them), and therefore the current lawsuit seems to a certain extent to be hypocritical. In our proposed approach, the USPS, as one of Armstrong's primary sponsors, would be responsible for his doping actions and as we explain below there could be a contract between athlete and sponsor preventing the sponsor from suing the athlete.

To recapitulate, we argue that the athlete's sponsoring organisations should become accountable for their athletes' actions, and take on the burden of proving that the athlete is not doping prior to and while sponsoring that athlete. In addition, the penalties for doping should not fall on the athlete and his/her team and doctors, but instead should fall solely on the athlete's sponsors. The penalties should also be severe enough to have a significant impact on the financial operations of the sponsoring organizations. Finally, we argue that WADA should still be responsible for its own testing for doping and enforcement of penalties. In this way, the payoff matrix that leads to sponsors unwittingly (or otherwise) sponsoring an athlete that uses illegal performance enhancing drugs ceases to hold sway over professional sports, and consequently, athletes would no longer have strong financial incentives to discount their future health in exchange for current improvements in performance.

Of course, we recognize that this shift in the burden of proof would not be easy to implement in practice. In particular, we identify three possible criticisms:

1) Many of the details of how this policy would be enforced remain unaddressed, including how often WADA conducts tests on athletes and whether these are planned or surprise tests, how often WADA updates its testing standards and whether it shares these standards with the sponsorship industry, and how multiple sponsors of the same athlete would conduct testing and how penalties would be assessed if their shared athlete was found to be doping.

2) This policy would seem to offer sponsorship companies even stronger reasons than those they currently have to sue any of their athletes found by WADA to be doping. The sponsorship company might argue, for example, that it cannot possibly monitor its athletes 24 hours per day, 365 days per year, and it had, to the best of its ability, monitored and tested the athlete who was now found to be doping. The sponsor would then argue that the athlete engaged in doping on his or her own accord, despite the sponsor's efforts to prevent doping, and the athlete is therefore at fault.

3) Sponsorship money enables professional sports to exist and be shared by millions of enthusiasts around the globe. Without sponsorship money, there would be no professional sport industry as we know it (and enjoy it) today.

We recognize the validity of the first criticism, and leave it open for discussion of possible solutions. Indeed, implementing this proposed approach would be complex, as it represents a major change to the status quo. The elements related to enforcement and testing that we mention are likely to be some of the more difficult and contentious implementation aspects of the proposed shift. As to the second possible criticism, since the sponsors would be held responsible for the actions of their athletes under the approach we propose, we suggest that the athlete-sponsor contract could be written to prevent such lawsuits, but this criticism remains open for further reflection, as some may want to argue that the athlete should be held at least co-responsible together with the sponsor for his/her actions, under the assumption that she/he is an autonomous subject making autonomous decisions. We would like to resist this solution of co-responsibility, though; as we and others have identified elsewhere, (King and Robeson 2007; King and Robeson 2013; Camporesi and McNamee 2014) athletes are often vulnerable subjects who find themselves at the centre of a payoff matrix which makes autonomous decisions very difficult if not impossible. We argue that the only way to break this payoff matrix leading to a "win at all costs attitude" and to incentives to doping is to hold only the sponsors responsible for the actions of their sponsored athletes.

Finally, while we are aware of the possibility that sponsors might withdraw significant money from the field of professional sport and of the consequences that such a withdrawal would have on the existence itself of professional sports, we think most sponsors would remain engaged in professional sport. The financial gains of product promotion would likely outweigh the costs of testing their athletes and being held accountable for their athletes' actions. In addition, sponsorship companies are already negatively affected by doping, (Straubel 2002) and therefore we think that they may be inclined to take up this idea if the proper international policy regime – including enforcement, testing, penalties, and positive incentives – were in place.

To conclude, the fields of sustainability and professional sport likely have much to gain from insightful comparisons, as both need to develop ethics and policy tools to alter the discounting of future good health (of the athlete, of the planet) in exchange for shorter-term returns (fame, sponsorship money, victory, economic gains). Currently, both athletes and the environment are being damaged as a result of a systematic, institutionalised payoff matrix that privileges shorter term gains over longer-term sustainability. The argument to shift the burden of proof that we propose here is a way to promote the long-term sustainability of professional sport by removing a key incentive for doping, and it draws on lessons learned from over twenty years of similar discussions in the environmental sustainability field. We can only hope that professional sport as an industry might succeed where environmental sustainability has up to now largely failed, and do so at a much quicker pace.

4.3 The case for research on enhancements

In this section I tackle the broader question of an ethical justification for research on enhancement or enhancement research (hence, ER). This question is surprisingly neglected in the bioethics literature on enhancement, as the leading critics of biomedical enhancement [Kass, Habermas, Annas, Fukuyama] have not addressed it directly. However, their statements against enhancement strongly suggest that research and development of enhancements would also be considered unethical from their point of view, on the basis of the argument that ER would promote an unethical practice, and should therefore be banned. However, I do not think that just because particular technologies aimed at enhancing human capacities are deemed to be not ethically permissible in a certain context, research on enhancement *per se* is also not ethically permissible. In this section I would like to start from this a reflection on the justifiability of ER in society.

To the best of my knowledge, the only authors that have raised the point about the necessity to establish a framework for, and to regulate, ER are Lev and co-authors (2010). They write:

> As with other biomedical interventions, research to assess the safety and efficacy of these enhancements in humans should be conducted before their introduction into clinical practice. (Lev, Miller, and Emanuel 2010, 101)

This is what should happen, but not what happens in practice. There is no system in place to regulate ER, and very little – if any – discussion about it. If this is the situation, it is also obvious that there are no safety precautions for the individuals who want to take on pharmacological enhancements, as there are no regulated trials that spell out the possible risks and harms, and benefits. Should this not be case? Or at least, should there not be a case for it? What could be the ethical justification for ER?

Lev and co-authors seem to justify research on enhancements on the basis of a health-related value:

> Categorically condemning research on biomedical enhancements as unethical is unwarranted, since at least some research on biomedical enhancements is likely to produce significant health benefits. Indeed, under certain circumstances enhancement research would be urgent, as it would address major public health concerns. Therefore, a blanket prohibition on enhancement research is unjustified. (Lev, Miller, and Emanuel 2010, 102)

While I agree with them that "a blanket prohibition on enhancement research is unjustified," it is not immediately clear that ER ought to be justified by having health-related social value, even though there might be some cases of "dual use" biomedical interventions, or interventions that can be used both as treatments and as enhancements. (Miller and Selgelid 2007) In such cases any health-related social value can be seen as an added value rather than a prerequisite. In all other cases, while the health of the research participant should of course still remain a primary concern, research on performance enhancing substances should have as its first epistemic goal the validity and reliability of performance enhancement claims. Of course this epistemic goal should be circumscribed by an ethical one, and thus the evaluation of risks and benefits needs to be modified when shifting from the clinical to the enhancement context[3]. Precisely what counts as benefit and risk in enhancement research need not be identical to what counts as benefit and risk in clinical research.

What policies would need to be put in place to regulate ER? To the best of my knowledge, the only existing analysis of the type of regulations that would need to be implemented has been carried out by US law and bioethics scholar Hank Greely (2011). Greely reviews the policy tools available in the US, and shows how not necessarily new regulatory frameworks or systems would have to be invented, since existing regulations could accommodate biomedical enhancements. (Greely 2011) This would happen because:

> FDA regulation already covers enhancements. If a firm were to seek approval to sell a new drug for enhancement purposes, no new safety regulation would be needed in the United States. The company would have to conduct serious clinical trials and to demonstrate to the satisfaction of the FDA that the drug was safe and effective for the intended use. (Greely 2011, 510)

Greely proceeds then to identify two main issues that would need careful consideration to assure the safety of enhancements, namely the regulation of off-label use of pharmaceuticals for enhancement purposes, and possibly the increased regulation of dietary supplements. As it is plausible to speculate,

---

3   For this argument I am indebted to Mike J McNamee (see Camporesi and Mc-Namee 2014).

many and probably the vast majority of biomedical enhancements would be approved to treat disease and used off-label as enhancements. The off-label practice of use for pharmaceuticals is already a widespread practice in the US, so from this point of view the introduction of enhancements would not be substantially new.

What is off-label use? In the US, after a drug's approval, the FDA works with the manufacturer to create a drug label that contains information about the drug, how it should be administered, and the indications for which it has been approved. Since the FDA itself does not regulate the practice of medicine, off-label use of FDA-approved drugs is a legal and common medical practice: after approval, a licensed doctor can use a drug for any indication he/she consider appropriate. (National Task Force on CME 2013) I find the widespread use of off-label drugs in the US very problematic from a scientific and ethical point of view, since patients can be prescribed drugs by doctors *without any evidential basis* that the drug works in a context different from the one for which it was tested in clinical trials. Greely seems to concur with me on this point when he writes that:

> Drugs can be approved as safe and effective for one use against one disease, based on clinical trial evidence, but then prescribed off-label for uses in people without that disease, or perhaps any disease, without any proof that the drug is either safe or effective for the prescribed use. (Greely 2011, 511)

Contrary to very strong libertarian thinking, I do not think that the current off-label system promotes autonomy by empowering the individual with freedom of choice (note that this is indeed the rhetoric underlying so many proponents of DTC advertising), but that the patient needs and deserves some protection from the market's free reign. While the "empowering freedom" argument could work in an ideal society, in practice the intricate financial ties between pharmaceutical companies, lobbies and politics in the US create markets where there is no legitimate demand, and lead to ethically problematic situations such as the case of prescriptions for Ritalin or Adderall for adults under the rubric of adult ADHD. (Wilens et al. 2008) For all these reasons, I do not think that the entry of enhancements in society through the "off-label" system would be desirable. It would be equivalent to entering society "through the back door" – to borrow an expression from Buchanan (2011) – as they are now. Once again that would happen without the appropriate regulation and demonstration of effectiveness and risks/harm data, and without any transparency, or accountability.

Another issue that needs to be taken into account when reflecting on the regulation of access of enhancements in society is the necessity to tighten up regulations regarding dietary supplements. In the US, regulation of such supplements is minimal according to the Dietary Supplement Health and Education Act (DSHEA 1994), which defines the FDA's power to regulate them. The manufacturer neither has to prove that the supplements are safe, nor that they are effective, in order to get approval to enter the market. On the contrary, the burden of proof rests on the FDA to prove to a court that a supplement is unsafe in order to remove it from the market. (Greely 2011) The only requirement for the manufacturer is that "that product label information is truthful and not misleading," and even that minimum requirement is often not respected. As a way of illustration of this trend, consider "think Gum," a chewing gum marketed in the US as a dietary supplement as the "brain boosting chewing gum."[4] According to the product website,[5] the chewing gum improves memory by 25 %, as demonstrated by a "peer reviewed study" (of course, there are no data on the peer-reviewed study whatsoever). It is interesting to note how the motto for the gum is "stop cheating, start chewing," therefore going contra one of the commonly raised arguments against using enhancements, namely that they are a way of cheating! The system in place for regulation of dietary supplements in the US seems therefore to be a very fruitful terrain for attempts to fraud scientifically or medically naïve individuals, in another instance of the 'sciencexploitation' phenomenon described by Caulfield (2011) and applied in section 3.2 to direct-to-consumer genetic tests to scout out children's talents. (Caulfield 2011; Camporesi 2013)

Therefore, it is plausible to speculate that biomedical enhancements which are manufactured as pills could also reach the market, at least in the US, as dietary supplements, therefore evading completely the purview of FDA. Even if they were marketed as pharmaceuticals to treat diseases, though, we

---

4   For this example I am also indebted to Greely (2011)

5   [http://thinkgum.com /] [accessed, July 18, 2014]

have seen how they could still be used off-label without having to demonstrate either the safety or the efficacy for that particular use. The possibility that pharmacological enhancement could enter the market in this way seems to me particularly worrisome. Instead, I think that a much better – and more accountable – way for enhancements to gain entry to society would be to put in place a regulatory system for clinical research, and for prescription of performance-enhancing substances outside the current disease (including off-label prescriptions) model.

In the next section I attempt to lay the ground for the discussion of how to shift the debate on enhancement technologies from the ethical level to a policy level. See (Camporesi and McNamee 2014) for a detailed discussion of the need to regulate the introduction of performance enhancing technologies in professional sports, which at the moment amounts to "unregulated clinical research" as defined by King and Robeson (2007).

4.4 A deliberative democracy approach to deal with moral disagreement in the bioethical debate

Is the enhancement debate satisfactorily answered with a discussion carried out at the ethical level? I start answering this question by analysing the original perspective put forward by Häyry in his book, *Rationality and the genetic challenge.*[6] (Häyry 2010) Häyry analyses three ways to deal with what he considers the challenges posed by genetics to society, which he refers to heuristically as neoconsequentialism, neo-virtue ethics, and neo-deontology. (Häyry 2010) A genetic challenge is defined as a "set of questions raised by the engineering of political and medical solutions to the original threats posed by nonhuman and human nature" to which "we cannot readily agree on what our reactions should be and on what grounds." (Häyry 2010, 2) As the subtitle of the book suggests, genetic challenges are understood as possible ways to "make people better." Häyry provides an extensive overview of the state of the field by analyzing seven case studies, namely, preimplantation genetic diagnosis

---

6   This section is a slightly revised form of the first half of a paper originally published on *Cambridge Quarterly of Healthcare Ethics* (2011): 20(2), 248-257, and co-authored with Paolo Maugeri.

(PGD), the possibility to design children, savior siblings, reproductive cloning, embryonic stem cell research, gene therapies, and considerable life extension techniques. As depicted by Häyry – even though such labeling may not be correct, as John Coggon and John Harris have suggested (Coggon 2011; Harris 2011) – the first framework ("neo-consequentialism" or "rational tangibility") focuses on persons and how they value life and is represented in the works of John Harris and Jonathan Glover; the second ("neo-virtue ethics" or "moral transcendence") puts the emphasis on traditions and is exemplified by Michael Sandel and Leon Kass; and the third ("neo-deontology") focuses on principles, with Jürgen Habermas and Ronald Green given as examples. Each of these frameworks reaches very different conclusions in terms of the ethical acceptability of the genetic challenges presented above. Although the central part of Häyry's book is devoted to the description of the state of the art concerning the seven wonders (or sins) of genetics, the most innovative chapter is the second, where Häyry spells out his methodological approach and the aim of the book. Häyry's original contribution to the discussion is the claim that it is not possible to argue with philosophical tools which of the three frameworks is best for assessing the ethical justifiability of a new biotechnological practice, as the three approaches differ in the fundamental values and principles they employ. Häyry tests the internal coherence of each position, and concludes that it is not possible to assess the superiority of any position over another on philosophical grounds. In his words:

> If different approaches (or rationalities or methods of genethics) cannot be universally graded and put into order, as I am saying, then conflicting normative views cannot be put into one rational order, either, and we have no philosophical way of telling once and for all whether we should or should not engage in procreative selection, reproductive or therapeutic cloning, genetic engineering, or considerable life extension. (Häyry 2010, 238)

According to this perspective, all ethical principles and judgments have respectable support if they meet the criteria of internal consistency and if in each case the combination of principles and judgments is a stable balance from the author's point of view (a so-called reflective equipoise). (Häyry 2010, 50) But, if Häyry's arguments are correct and ethical theories cannot be pre-

ferred on rational grounds, what are we readers left to do with his polite bystander view? As Häyry himself puts it: "Do we have any role in genethics, if
all this [the content of the book] is to be believed?" (Häyry 2010, 238) In the
last pages of the book, he lays out the work for the philosophically informed
readers, when he writes that there are at least 72 stances that could be critically
examined by the philosopher, resulting from the multiplication of three viable
methods of ethics, three normative strands, and eight topics. (Häyry 2010,
239) We do not think that focusing our attention on such a nonconfrontational experience would necessarily be an improvement over the actual state
of the field and over the recognition of the existence of moral disagreement
concerning questions raised by the genetic challenges. What should we do
with Häyry's nonconfrontationalism then? Should we take it as a claim about
diverse methods in ethics, or rather as an insightful plea to confront views at
another, more appropriate level? We think that confrontational ethics is still
important in many respects and that, if properly framed, can inform debates
and, hopefully, help at reaching the right conclusions.

Moral disagreement in society will persist, no matter what philosophers
may say. This, however, is not an indication of the fact that all views in the
field of philosophical ethics are equivalent or incommensurable. Rather, it
highlights how, in practice, we face a political problem. The pressing questions
posed by genethics do not allow us simply to acknowledge that moral positions differ and then nonconfrontationally to concern ourselves with ironing
out internal inconsistencies. Instead, they demand a shift in focus from classical philosophical ethics to the realm of political philosophy. Writes Häyry:

> Philosophical considerations can show that some arguments are flawed and
> others open to discussion, but they cannot prove to everybody's satisfaction
> the rightness or wrongness of selection, cloning, or new treatments. (Häyry
> 2010, 238)

In this passage Häyry is conflating two issues that should be kept distinct
for analytical purposes. One issue is whether philosophical considerations, or
arguments, can prove the rightness of anything at all. Quite another is whether
they can prove it to everybody's satisfaction. The first is a question about moral
relativism, the second one of political pluralism, that is, the claim that there

exist different, and sometimes hard to reconcile, values in society. Let us tackle the first problem first. If Häyry's main claim were about moral relativism, then there would be several ways to spell it out that he does not attempt in his book. For instance, why is it impossible to say that something, say one of the genetic challenges, is ethically justifiable or not? Is it because there is no such thing as objective moral truth? Or, more simply, is it that, even if objective morality existed, it would be unreachable by ethical thinking? Whereas the former would be an ontological claim, the latter would be an epistemological one. Häyry's position seems to be orthogonal to all these options. What he really seems to say is that there are different ways of doing ethics, none of them being illegitimate, at least as long as they are internally consistent and in some accordance with how things are in the world. As Coggon puts it, "a claim in support of simultaneous, non exclusive, yet competing rationality is a claim about the rightness of pluralism in ethics." (Coggon 2011, 50) Accepting Häyry's position may mean that each of the three methods he outlines has contradictory claims that cannot be undermined by other approaches, thus giving rise to irresolvable disagreement. For example, does the fact that Sandel/Kass-like conclusions are drawn by appeals to traditional values render them invulnerable to critiques by the rational tangibility approach of Harris and Glover and vice versa?

As for the second issue we mentioned, namely, political pluralism, the absence of agreement on a particular issue poses the question of how to reach a reasonable consensus, even if provisional or revisable, in the *polis*. People may maintain their private rationalities (or rational moralities) on the basis of philosophical arguments, but reasonable people may think that it is still worthwhile to reach a consensus in order to make decisions at the policy level. The question at stake, therefore, is not so much one of politeness (referring to the polite bystander view proposed by Häyry) but is one of indicating at what level each kind of rationality can effectively prove insightful and, as a consequence, at what level confrontations should take place.

The genetic challenges as described by Häyry are public questions requiring, ideally, public answers. It is in this regard that we do not see Häyry's "polite bystander" approach as exhaustive. Practical questions such as who should decide on ethical issues related to genetic technologies cannot be answered solely by reference to internally consistent rationalities. On the contrary, we think that, by following the route indicated by Häyry, we run the risk of ending up with a cornucopia of ethical perspectives, each internally consistent but providing mere philosophical amusement. If genetic challenges are to be taken seriously, as concrete instances of moral disagreement in the real world, then certain real-world questions concerning whose interests are challenged and how these can reasonably be reconciled cannot be escaped or masked behind the polite facade of a nonconfrontational notion of rationality. At least three levels ought to be distinguished here:

1) the nonconfrontational philosophical level described by Häyry, which is useful for assessing the internal consistency of each ethical position;

2) the confrontational philosophical level, which takes into account other ethical perspectives (after they have been assessed for consistency with the first approach);

3) the decision-making political level, in which moral disagreement is dealt with in practice.

As an alternative to the polite bystander approach, we suggest that the problem of "everybody's satisfaction" could be better addressed by engaging the different ethical perspectives in a process of public reason giving in the spirit of deliberative democracy (DD), as defined by Gutmann and Thompson (Gutmann and Thompson 2004) and applied to genethics issues by Farrelly. (Farrelly 2009) On this view, "first-order" theories are ethical perspectives that seek to resolve moral disagreement by demonstrating that alternative theories and principles should be rejected. First-order theories "measure their success by whether they resolve the conflict consistently on their own term. Their aim is to be the single theory that resolves moral disagreement." (Gutmann and Thompson 2004, 126) In Häyry's book, first-order theories can be assimilated to the three ways he describes to deal with the genetic challenges. Whereas Häyry's polite bystander view claims that the validity of first-order theories should be assessed only internally and not confronting one theory with another, a fruitful way forward in the discussion of the genetic challenge is a second-order theory approach, which deals with the moral disagreement residual of first-order theories. DD seeks a resolution to the moral disagreement by adopting a dynamic conception of political justification, which is both morally and politically provisional. (Gutmann and Thompson 2004, 132) Within this DD perspective, the resolution of first-order moral disagreement needs to respect the DD principles of reciprocity, publicity, and accountability and seeks a mutually binding (though provisional, therefore, at a specific time) decision, on the basis of mutually justifiable reasons. Such a DD approach is not morally neutral, nor does it claim to be. Indeed, the quality of moral neutrality is both undesirable and unattainable according to Gutmann and Thompson. If we accept this direction, we could read Häyry's polite bystander view as a claim about first order theories, to which we could add as a further step our steering toward the realm of political philosophy. How can a second-order DD approach build on the confrontational analysis of first-order theories applied to genetic enhancements in sports that we discussed above? The details of this process in the context of decision-making in sports would, of course, need to be spelled out in practice, but in this regard we can say that the current process of decision-making in sports is unsatisfactory at best.

Consider, for example, the ruling made by the International Association of Athletics Federations (IAAF) concerning the admissibility of the runner Caster Semenya to compete with women after charging her of not belonging properly to the category, which was neither transparent nor respectful of her privacy. (Camporesi and Maugeri 2010; Karkazis et al. 2012) Furthermore, the reasons for Semenya's banning and subsequent readmission were never made public, though not respecting the criteria of publicity that is fundamental in the DD approach. In the context of decisions surrounding the ethical justifiability of a gene enhancement (or other kind of enhancement) practice in sports, we envisage a DD process that gives reasons to all the moral constituents involved in the field, where moral constituents is understood as all "those who are in effect bound by the decision, even though they may not have [but maybe they should have, as we argue] a voice in making them," (Gutmann and Thompson 2004, 135) therefore including at least, but not only, the athletes.

To recapitulate, Häyry identifies three competing approaches used by scholars in the debate on the ethics of genetic technologies (what he refers to as "genethics"): consequentialism; teleology or virtue-ethics and deontology. (Häyry 2010) Häyry argues that these three approaches are "incommensurable" because they respectively define (a) utility; (b) human flourishing or well-being; and (c) persons as the entities that matter in the ethical debate. Häyry also argues that in practice the ethical judgments about the ethical permissibility of a technology depend ultimately on the choice of world-views, attitudes and ideas about what counts in the moral discussion. Therefore, if we do not agree on the "unit of measurement" itself of discussion, then it will be impossible to actually compare the outcomes of discussions grounded in different approaches. For Häyry, the three approaches can all be simultaneously valid, and the only necessary condition for their validity is that they are internally coherent/consistent. The only role for the philosopher in this field is to adopt a "polite bystander" role and assess the internal consistency/coherency of each account. Rather than adopting a "polite bystander" view, I think that a more productive way forward in the discussion of gen-ethics could be based on a "moderate pluralistic approach to public health policy and ethics" as the one delineated by Selgelid (2009, 2012) coupled with a DD approach as the one spelled out by Gutmann and Thompson (2004), and aimed at reaching publicly shared decisions about the acceptability of a particular technology.

Indeed, often individuals' motivations for seeking enhancements are that they see them as positional goods, able to give them a competitive advantage. Therefore, the differential access to enhancement technologies is likely to exacerbate the existing inequalities in society. Along similar lines to what is done by Häyry, Selgelid spells out the three main approaches used in the enhancement debate to try to – unsuccessfully – resolve controversies regarding the particular application of an enhancement technology. He refers to the three approaches as utilitarianism, egalitarianism, and libertarianism. (Selgelid 2012; Selgelid 2013) As each perspective tends to place absolute or overriding weight on the values they emphasize (respectively utility, equality, and liberty), consequently the current approach to the enhancement debate is not able to make any substantial progress. To obviate the current misbalance in debate between the value of liberty and other important values (such as equality and utility), Selgelid argues in favour of a contextual approach that spells out, and tries to balance between, the values by shifting the focus of the debate on enhancement towards the analysis of how to reach a "fair" trade-off between the different values. What would Selgelid's moderate pluralistic approach entail in practice? First, it would start with the aim to promote the three values of liberty, equality and utility as independently legitimate social goals, without any of them being by default overriding the other. Secondly, it would aim to strike a balance and make trade-offs between the values in cases where they conflict, with the assumption that no value has priority over the others. (Selgelid 2009) Selgelid also argues that the only possible way to make tangible progress in the enhancement debate is to address the controversial issues through a rigorous empirical analysis and a case by case contextual approach, which is what I tried to do in this work. Therefore, for Selgelid, the way to resolve disputes about enhancement is not the polite-bystander view to which the philosopher is relegated as suggested by Häyry, but a fourth approach, which he refers to as a "moderate pluralistic approach to public health policy and ethics."

One potential problem with Selgelid's moderate pluralistic approach is the apparent incommensurability of the values of liberty, equality and utility. Hence, questions such as "How much utility overweighs how much liberty (or vice versa) in a particular case?" seem impossible to answer. Selgelid is aware of this issue, which may be irresolvable from a general, abstract philosophical viewpoint of comparing first order theories. Not so, however, when the level of analysis is shifted to the policy-making level, and when decisions need to be taken regarding the ethical acceptability of a particular technology, and the ethically justifiability limits – for example – on personal liberty in favour of equality or on equality in favour of utility and so on and so forth. This is where the DD approach comes into place.

On this DD view, "first-order" ethical frameworks (i.e. deontology, utilitarianism, virtue ethics; or libertarianism, egalitarianism and utilitariasnism) try to resolve moral disagreement regarding a particular technology by demonstrating why that particular ethical theory is superior to another. This approach anyway is deemed to fail since, as pointed out by Häyry, different ethical frameworks are incommensurable as they use different "unit-values" (person, utility, wellbeing or human-flourishing, etc.), and the choice of which ethical framework to adopt in the first place is guided by the preference of the individual for one "unit-value" over another. Notwithstanding the impossibility to reach a moral agreement with first order theories, individuals who adopt different approaches may still agree that questions raised by the intersection of genetics and society demand public answer, and therefore that confrontation needs to take place at the societal and public level. The DD approach deals with the moral disagreement residual of first-order theories and seeks a resolution by adopting a dynamic conception of political justification.

This second order approach aims at reaching a mutually binding (to all parties involved) consensus achieved through principles of reciprocity, publicity, and accountability on mutually justifiable reasons. (Gutmann and Thompson 2004) The consensus reached would be provisional, and subject to revision, depending on the consequences of the policy applications. For example, in the case of research on enhancements, it could be revised depending on the extent of the black market of pharmaceutical for enhancement purposes (which is at the moment a widespread problem for the case of Ritalin and Adderall).

Bibliography

Abrahams, Adolphe. 1958. "The Use and Abuse of Drugs by Athletes." *Addiction* 55 (1) (July): 23–28. doi:10.1111/j.1360-0443.1958.tb05458.x.

Adams, Stephen. 2012. "British couples flying to US for banned baby sex selection," *The Telegraph* http://www.telegraph.co.uk/health/healthnews/9504503/British-couples-flying-to-US-for-banned-baby-sex-selection.html

"Adenosine Deaminase Deficiency." 2013. *Genetics Home Reference*. Accessed August 12. http://ghr.nlm.nih.gov/condition/adenosine-deaminase-deficiency.

Agar, Nicholas. 2008. *Liberal Eugenics: In Defence of Human Enhancement*. Malden, MA: Blackwell Pub.

Agassi, Andre. 2010. *Open: an Autobiography*. New York: Vintage Books.

Aiuti, Alessandro, Federica Cattaneo, Stefania Galimberti, Ulrike Benninghoff, Barbara Cassani, Luciano Callegaro, Samantha Scaramuzza, et al. 2009. "Gene Therapy for Immunodeficiency Due to Adenosine Deaminase Deficiency." *New England Journal of Medicine* 360 (5) (January 29): 447–458. doi:10.1056/NEJMoa0805817.

Allhoff, Fritz, Patrick Lin, and Jesse Steinberg. 2010. "Ethics of Human Enhancement: An Executive Summary." *Science and Engineering Ethics* 17 (2): 201–212. doi:10.1007/s11948-009-9191-9.

Archard, David. 2004. *Children: Rights and Childhood*. 2nd ed. London ; New York: Routledge.

Arendt, Hannah. 1958. *The Human Condition*. Chicago [etc.]: The University of Chicago Press.

Atry, A., Hansson, M. G., & Kihlbom, U. 2011. Gene Doping and the Responsibility of Bioethicists. Sport, Ethics and Philosophy, 5(2), 149-160.

Atry, A., Hansson, M. G., & Kihlbom, U. 2012. Beyond the Individual:

Sources of Attitudes Towards Rule Violation in Sport. Sport, Ethics and Philosophy, 6(4), 467-479.

Atry, A. 2013. Transforming the Doping Culture: Whose responsibility, what responsibility? http://www.diva-portal.org/smash/record.jsf?pid=diva2:644734

Baoutina, Anna, Ian E Alexander, John E J Rasko, and Kerry R Emslie. 2008. "Developing Strategies for Detection of Gene Doping." *The Journal of Gene Medicine* 10 (1) (January): 3–20. doi:10.1002/jgm.1114.

Barinaga, M. 1999. "BIOTECH PATENTS:Genentech, UC Settle Suit for $200 Million." *Science* 286 (5445) (November 26): 1655a–1655. doi:10.1126/science.286.5445.1655a.

Bartlett, Jason. 2003. "Mighty Mice Hold Hope for Muscle Ailments." *Penn Current Nes.* http://www.upenn.edu/pennnews/current/node/2215.

Barton-Davis, E R, D I Shoturma, A Musaro, N Rosenthal, and H L Sweeney. 1998. "Viral Mediated Expression of Insulin-like Growth Factor I Blocks the Aging-related Loss of Skeletal Muscle Function." *Proceedings of the National Academy of Sciences of the United States of America* 95 (26) (December 22): 15603–15607.

Baruch, Susannah, David Kaufman, and Kathy L Hudson. 2008. "Genetic Testing of Embryos: Practices and Perspectives of US in Vitro Fertilization Clinics." *Fertility and Sterility* 89 (5) (May): 1053–1058. doi:10.1016/j.fertnstert.2007.05.048.

Baumann, Gerhard P. 2012. "Growth Hormone Doping in Sports: a Critical Review of Use and Detection Strategies." *Endocrine Reviews* 33 (2) (April): 155–186. doi:10.1210/er.2011-1035.

Baumgartner, I. 2000. "Therapeutic Angiogenesis: Theoretic Problems Using Vascular Endothelial Growth Factor." *Current Cardiology Reports* 2 (1) (January): 24–28.

BBC News Health. 2013. "'Test-tube Baby' Brown Hails Pioneers on 35th Birthday." *BBC News Health*, July 25. http://www.bbc.co.uk/news/health-23448665.

Beauchamp, Tom L., and James F. Childress. 2001. *Principles of Biomedical Ethics*. 5th ed. New York, N.Y: Oxford University Press.

Beier, HM, and JO Beckham. 1991. "Implications and Consequences of the

German Embryo Protection Act." *Human Reproduction* 6 (4): 607–608.

Biondi, Stefano. 2013. "Access to Medical-assisted Reproduction and PGD in Italian Law: a Deadly Blow to an Illiberal Statute? Commentary to the European Court on Human Rights's Decision Costa and Pavan v Italy (ECtHR, 28 August 2012, App. 54270/2010)." *Medical Law Review* (April 3). doi:10.1093/medlaw/fwt010.

Blake, Matt. 2012. "Torture or Training? Inside the Brutal Chinese Gymnasium Where the Country's Future Olympic Stars Are Beaten into Shape." *The Daily Mail*, August 1. http://www.dailymail.co.uk/news/article-2182127/How-China-trains-children-win-gold--standing-girls-legs-young-boys-hang-bars.html.

Bond, David. 2013. "Jamaica Doping Scandals Tip of Iceberg, Says Senior Drug Tester." *BBC News*, November 11. http://www.bbc.co.uk/sport/0/athletics/24900565.

Borrione, P, A Mastrone, R A Salvo, A Spaccamiglio, L Grasso, and A Angeli. 2008. "Oxygen Delivery Enhancers: Past, Present, and Future." *Journal of Endocrinological Investigation* 31 (2) (February): 185–192.

Bortolotti, Lisa. 2010. *Delusions and Other Irrational Beliefs*. International Perspectives in Philosophy and Psychiatry. Oxford ; New York: Oxford University Press.

Bortolotti, Lisa, and Daniela Cutas. 2009. "Reproductive and Parental Autonomy: An Argument for Compulsory Parental Education." *Reproductive Biomedicine Online* 19 Suppl 1: 5–14.

Bortolotti, Lisa, and John Harris. 2006. "Disability, Enhancement and the Harm-benefit Continuum." In *Freedom and Responsibility in Reproductive Choice*, edited by John R. Spencer and Antje Du Bois-Pedain, 31–49. Oxford ; Portland, Or: Hart Pub.

Bostrom, Nick, and Sandberg, Anders. 2007. "The Wisdom of Nature: An Evolutionary Heuristic for Human Enhancement." In *Enhancement of Human Beings*. Oxford: Oxford University Press.

Breivik, Harald, Beverly Collett, Vittorio Ventafridda, Rob Cohen, and Derek Gallacher. 2006. "Survey of Chronic Pain in Europe: Prevalence, Impact on Daily Life, and Treatment." *European Journal of Pain (London, England)* 10 (4) (May): 287–333. doi:10.1016/j.ejpain.2005.06.009.

Broberg, Gunnar, and Nils Roll-Hansen. 2005. *Eugenics and the Welfare State:*

Sterilization Policy in Denmark, Sweden, Norway, and Finland. Rev. pbk. ed. East Lansing: Michigan State University Press.

Brooks, M Alison, and Beth A Tarini. 2011. "Genetic Testing and Youth Sports." *JAMA: The Journal of the American Medical Association* 305 (10) (March 9): 1033–1034. doi:10.1001/jama.2011.286.

Buchanan, Allen. 2009. "Human Nature and Enhancement." *Bioethics* 23 (3): 141–150. doi:10.1111/j.1467-8519.2008.00633.x.

———. 2011. *Beyond Humanity? : the Ethics of Biomedical Enhancement*. Oxford: Oxford University Press.

Buchanan, Allen E, Dan Brock, Norman Daniels, and Daniel Wikler. 2000. *From Chance to Choice: Genetics and Justice*. Cambridge, U.K.; New York: Cambridge University Press.

Bury, Liz. 2013. "Lance Armstrong Faces Lawsuit over Lies in Memoirs." *The Guardian*, August 9. http://www.theguardian.com/books/2013/aug/09/lance-armstrong-lawsuit-lies-memoirs-compensation.

Calfee, R., and P. Fadale. 2006. "Popular Ergogenic Drugs and Supplements in Young Athletes." *PEDIATRICS* 117 (3) (March 1): e577–e589. doi:10.1542/peds.2005-1429.

Camporesi, Silvia and Lisa Bortolotti. 2008. "Reproductive Cloning in Humans and Therapeutic Cloning in Primates: Is the Ethical Debate Catching up with the Recent Scientific Advances?" *Journal of Medical Ethics* 34 (9) (September): e15. doi:10.1136/jme.2007.023879.

Camporesi, Silvia. 2010. "Choosing Deafness with Preimplantation Genetic Diagnosis: An Ethical Way to Carry on a Cultural Bloodline?" *Cambridge Quarterly of Healthcare Ethics: CQ: The International Journal of Healthcare Ethics Committees* 19 (1): 86–96. doi:10.1017/S0963180109990272.

———. 2013. "Bend It Like Beckham! The Ethics of Genetically Testing Children for Athletic Potential." *Sport, Ethics and Philosophy* 7 (2) (May): 175–185. doi:10.1080/17511321.2013.780183.

Camporesi, Silvia, and James A. Knuckles. 2014. "Shifting the Burden of Proof in Doping: Lessons from Environmental Sustainability Applied to High-Performance Sport." *Reflective Practice*. 15(1), 106-118, 10.1080/14623943.2013.869203

Camporesi, Silvia, and Paolo Maugeri. 2010. "Caster Semenya: Sport, Categories and the Creative Role of Ethics." *Journal of Medical Ethics* 36:

378–379.

———. 2011. "Genetic Enhancement in Sports: The Role of Reason and Private Rationalities in the Public Arena." *Cambridge Quarterly of Healthcare Ethics* 20 (02): 248–257. doi:10.1017/S0963180110000897.

Camporesi, Silvia, and M J McNamee. 2014. "Performance Enhancement, Elite Athletes and Anti Doping Governance: Comparing Human Guinea Pigs in Pharmaceutical Research and Professional Sports." *Philosophy, Ethics and Humanities in Medicine.* (9)4, doi: 10.1186/1747-5341-9-4.

———. 2013. "Is There a Role for Genetic Testing in Sports?" In *eLS*, edited by John Wiley & Sons, Ltd. Chichester, UK: John Wiley & Sons, Ltd. http://doi.wiley.com/10.1002/9780470015902.a0024203.

———. 2012. "Gene Transfer for Pain: A Tool to Cope with the Intractable, or an Unethical Endurance-enhancing Technology?" *Life Sciences, Society and Policy Journal* 8 (1): 20–31.

Cassata, Francesco. 2011. *Building the New Man: Eugenics, Racial Science and Genetics in Twentieth-century Italy.* Translated by Erin O'Loughlin. CEU Press Studies in the History of Medicine v. 3. Budapest ; New York: Central European University Press.

Cassell, Eric J. 2004. *The Nature of Suffering and the Goals of Medicine.* 2nd ed. New York: Oxford University Press.

Catlin, D H, and T H Murray. 1996. "Performance-enhancing Drugs, Fair Competition, and Olympic Sport." *JAMA: The Journal of the American Medical Association* 276 (3) (July 17): 231–237.

Caulfield, Timothy. 2011. "Predictive or Preposterous? The Marketing of DTC Genetic Testing." *Journal of Science Communication* 10 (03): C02.

Chan, Sarah, and John Harris. 2008. "In Support of Human Enhancement." *Studies in Ethics, Law, and Technology* 1 (1) (January 8). doi:10.2202/1941-6008.1007. http://www.degruyter.com/view/j/selt.2007.1.1/selt.2007.1.1.1007/selt.2007.1.1.1007.xml.

Chang, Emily. 2009. "In China, DNA Tests on Kids ID Genetic Gifts, Careers." *CNN News* (August 5). http://edition.cnn.com/2009/WORLD/asiapcf/08/03/china.dna.children.ability/.

Charon, Rita, and Martha Montello. 2002. *Stories Matter: The Role of Narrative in Medical Ethics.* Reflective Bioethics. New York: Routledge.

Cintado, Ana. 2007. "Eating Disorders and Gymnastics." In *Women and Sports in the United States: a Documentary Reader*, edited by Jean O'Reilly and Susan K. Cahn. Boston: Northeastern University Press.

Clinicaltrials.gov. 2014a. "Search on Clinicaltrials.gov for 'Gene Transfer AND Pain'." Accessed March 19. http://www.clinicaltrials.gov/ct2/resu lts?term=gene+transfer+pain&Search=Search

———. 2014b. "Clinical Trial NCT00304837." Accessed March 19, 2014. http://clinicaltrials.gov/ct2/show/NCT00304837?term=gene+transfer +AND+pain&rank=3.

CNN Associated Press. 2007. "Track Star Marion Jones Pleads Guilty to Doping Deception." *CNN*, October 5. http://edition.cnn.com/2007/ US/10/05/jones.doping/.

Coggon, John. 2011. "Confrontations in 'Genethics': Rationalities, Challenges, and Methodological Responses." *Cambridge Quarterly of Healthcare Ethics* 20 (01) (January 11): 46–55. doi:10.1017/ S0963180110000617.

Cohen, I. Glenn. 2012. "HOW TO REGULATE MEDICAL TOURISM (AND WHY IT MATTERS FOR BIOETHICS): How to Regulate Medical Tourism." *Developing World Bioethics* 12 (1) (April): 9–20. doi:10.1111/j.1471-8847.2012.00317.x.

Cole, Phillip. 2007. "The Body Politic: Theorising Disability and Impairment." *Journal of Applied Philosophy* 24 (2): 169–176. doi:10.1111/ j.1468-5930.2007.00369.x.

Connor, Steve. 2013 Medical ethicist: Ban on sex selection of IVF embryos is not justified. *The Independent.* http://www.independent.co.uk/news/ science/medical-ethicist-ban-on-sex-selection-of-ivf-embryos-is-not-justified-8683940.html (accessed March 18, 2014)

Cooper, David. 1995. "Technology: Liberation or Enslavement?" In *Philosophy and Technology*, edited by Roger Fellows, 8–17. Royal Institute of Philosophy Supplement 38. Cambridge ; New York: Cambridge University Press.

Costanza, Andrade, Antunes, den Belt M, Boersma, Boesch, Catarino, et al. 1998. "Principles for Sustainable Governance of the Oceans." *Science (New York, N.Y.)* 281 (5374): 198–199.

Crust, Lee. 2007. "Mental Toughness in Sport: A Review." *International Journal of Sport and Exercise Psychology* 5 (3) (January): 270–290. doi:10.1080/1612

197X.2007.9671836.

Daiji World. 2013. "WADA Optimistic About Gene-doping Detection Research." *Daiji World*, June 7. http://www.daijiworld.com/news/news_disp.asp?n_id=176056.

Dahl, E. 2004. The presumption in favour of liberty: a comment on the HFEA's public consultation on sex selection. *Reproductive BioMedicine Online*, 8(3), 266-267.

Daniels, Norman. 2000. "Normal Functioning and the Treatment-enhancement Distinction." *Cambridge Quarterly of Healthcare Ethics: CQ: The International Journal of Healthcare Ethics Committees* 9 (3): 309–322.

Davis, Dena S. 1997. "Genetic Dilemmas and the Child's Right to an Open Future." *The Hastings Center Report* 27 (2) (March): 7. doi:10.2307/3527620.

De Melo-Martin, Immaculada. 2010. "Defending Human Enhancement Technologies: Unveiling Normativity." *Journal of Medical Ethics* 36 (8) (July 27): 483–487. doi:10.1136/jme.2010.036095.

DeGrazia, David. 2012. *Creation Ethics Genetics, Reproduction, and Quality of Life*. New York: Oxford University Press. http://lib.myilibrary.com?id=380775.

Deonandan, R., & Bente, A. 2014. "Assisted Reproduction and Cross-Border Maternal Surrogacy Regulations in Selected Nations". *British Journal of Medicine & Medical Research*, 4(1).

Dixon, Nicholas. 2007. "Sport, Parental Autonomy, and Children's Right to an Open Future." *Journal of the Philosophy of Sport* 34 (2): 147–159. doi:10.1080/00948705.2007.9714718.

Dolgin, Elie. 2010. "Fluctuating Baseline Pain Implicated in Failure of Clinical Trials." *Nature Medicine* 16 (10) (October): 1053–1053. doi:10.1038/nm1010-1053a.

Dorr, Gregory Michael. 2011. "Protection or Control? Women's Health, Sterilization Abuse, and Relf V. Weinberger." In *A Century of Eugenics in America: From the Indiana Experiment to the Human Genome Era*, edited by Paul A. Lombardo, 161–190. Bioethics and the Humanities. Bloomington, Ind: Indiana University Press.

Dorr, Gregory Michael, and Angela Logan. 2011. "'Quality, Not Mere Quantity, Counts': Black Eugenics and the NAACP Baby Contests." In

A Century of Eugenics in America: From the Indiana Experiment to the Human Genome Era, edited by Paul A. Lombardo, 68–92. Bioethics and the Humanities. Bloomington, Ind: Indiana University Press.

Douglas, Thomas. 2007. "Enhancement in Sport, and Enhancement Outside Sport." *Studies in Ethics, Law, and Technology* 1 (1) (January 21). doi:10.2202/1941-6008.1000. http://www.degruyter.com/view/j/selt.2007.1.1/selt.2007.1.1.1000/selt.2007.1.1.1000.xml.

Easley, Jason. 2013. "California Prisons Illegally Sterilized Hundreds of Female Inmates." *Politicus USA*, July 7. http://www.politicususa.com/2013/07/07/california-prisons-illegally-sterilized-hundreds-female-inmates.html.

ECHR. 2012. *CASE OF COSTA AND PAVAN V. ITALY*. European Court of Human Rights. http://hudoc.echr.coe.int/sites/eng/pages/search.aspx?i=001-112993#{"itemid":["001-112993"]} (accessed March 18, 2014)

Elliott, Carl. 2009. "What's Wrong with Enhancement Technology?" In *Readings in the Philosophy of Technology*, edited by Kaplan, David, 2nd edition, 431–442. Rowman & Littlefield Publishers.

Epstein, David J. 2013. *The Sports Gene: Inside the Science of Extraordinary Athletic Performance*. New York: Current.

Ethics Committee of the American Society of Reproductive Medicine. 2004. "Sex Selection and Preimplantation Genetic Diagnosis." *Fertility and Sterility* 82 Suppl 1 (September): S245–248. doi:10.1016/j.fertnstert.2004.05.016.

Eynon, Nir, Jonatan R Ruiz, José Oliveira, José Alberto Duarte, Ruth Birk, and Alejandro Lucia. 2011. "Genes and Elite Athletes: a Roadmap for Future Research." *The Journal of Physiology* 589 (Pt 13) (July 1): 3063–3070. doi:10.1113/jphysiol.2011.207035.

Fantz, Ashley. 2010. "The Next Frontier in Athletic Doping -- Genes." *CNN*. http://edition.cnn.com/2010/HEALTH/02/19/genetic.doping/index.html.

Farrelly, Colin. 2009. "Preimplantation Genetic Diagnosis, Reproductive Freedom, and Deliberative Democracy." *The Journal of Medicine and Philosophy* 34 (2) (April): 135–154. doi:10.1093/jmp/jhp016.

Feinberg, Joel. 1980a. "The Child's Right to an Open Future." In *Whose*

Child?: Children's Rights, Parental Authority, and State Power, edited by William Aiken and Hugh LaFollette. Totowa, N.J.: Littlefield, Adams.

———. 1980b. *Rights, Justice, and the Bounds of Liberty: Essays in Social Philosophy*. Princeton Series of Collected Essays. Princeton, N.J: Princeton University Press.

Fineschi, V, M Neri, and E Turillazzi. 2005. "The New Italian Law on Assisted Reproduction Technology (Law 40/2004)." *Journal of Medical Ethics* 31 (9) (September): 536–539. doi:10.1136/jme.2004.010231.

Freedman, B. 1987. "Equipoise and the Ethics of Clinical Research." *The New England Journal of Medicine* 317 (3) (July 16): 141–145. doi:10.1056/NEJM198707163170304.

Frieden, Terry. 2013. "Lance Armstrong Sued by U.S. for Post Office Sponsorship Funds." *CNN*, April 24. http://edition.cnn.com/2013/04/23/justice/justice-case-armstrong.

Fry, J. 2006. "Pain, Suffering and Paradox in Sport and Religion." In *Pain and Injury in Sport: Social and Ethical Analysis*, edited by Sigmund Loland, Berit Skirstad, and Ivan Waddington, 246–259. Ethics and Sport. London ; New York: Routledge.

Fukuyama, Francis. 2003. *Our Posthuman Future : Consequences of the Biotechnology Revolution*. New York: Picador.

Galton, Sir Francis. 1906. *Essays in Eugenics*. Honolulu, HI: University Press of the Pacific.

Gaspar, H. B. 2012. "Gene Therapy for ADA-SCID: Defining the Factors for Successful Outcome." *Blood* 120 (18) (November 1): 3628–3629. doi:10.1182/blood-2012-08-446559.

Giacca, M, and S Zacchigna. 2012. "VEGF Gene Therapy: Therapeutic Angiogenesis in the Clinic and Beyond." *Gene Therapy* 19 (6) (June): 622–629. doi:10.1038/gt.2012.17.

Giordano, Simona. 2010. *Exercise and Eating Disorders: An Ethical and Legal Analysis*. 1st ed. Ethics and Sport. London ; New York: Routledge.

Glover, Jonathan. 1992. "Future People, Disability and Screening." In *Justice Between Age Groups and Generations*, 429–44. New Haven, CT: Yale University Press.

———. 2007. *Choosing Children: Genes, Disability, and Design*. Oxford; New York: Clarendon Press.

Goins, William F, Justus B Cohen, and Joseph C Glorioso. 2012. "Gene Therapy for the Treatment of Chronic Peripheral Nervous System Pain." *Neurobiology of Disease* 48 (2) (November): 255–270. doi:10.1016/j.nbd.2012.05.005.

Gottweis, Herbert. 2002. "Stem Cell Policies in the United States and in Germany. Between Bioethics and Regulation." *Policy Studies Journal* 30 (4) (November): 444–469. doi:10.1111/j.1541-0072.2002.tb02158.x.

Grant, Bob. 2013. "Genetics Firm Gets Baby-Predicting Patent." *The Scientist*, October 4. http://www.the-scientist.com/?articles.view/articleNo/37781/title/Genetics-Firm-Gets-Baby-Predicting-Patent/.

Greely, Hank T. 2011. "Of Nails and Hammers: Human Biological Enhancement and U.S. Policy Tools." In *Enhancing Human Capacities*, edited by Julian Savulescu, R. H. J. ter Meulen, and Guy Kahane, 503–520. Chichester, West Sussex, U.K. ; Malden, MA: Wiley-Blackwell.

Gregory, Ted. 1996. "No Pain, No Fame: Line Blurry Between Playing, Paying." *The Chicago Tribune*, June 28. http://articles.chicagotribune.com/1996-07-28/sports/9607280254_1_pain-kerri-strug-gymnastics.

Gucciardi, Daniel F., Sandy Gordon, and James A. Dimmock. 2009. "Advancing Mental Toughness Research and Theory Using Personal Construct Psychology." *International Review of Sport and Exercise Psychology* 2 (1) (March): 54–72. doi:10.1080/17509840802705938.

Gutmann, Amy, and Dennis Thompson. 2004. *Why Deliberative Democracy?* Princeton, N.J: Princeton University Press.

Habermas, Jürgen. 2003. *The Future of Human Nature*. Cambridge, UK: Polity.

Haisma, H. J., and O. de Hon. 2006. "Gene Doping." *International Journal of Sports Medicine* 27 (4) (April): 257–266. doi:10.1055/s-2006-923986.

Hamilton, Tyler. 2012. *The Secret Race: Inside the Hidden World of the Tour de France: Doping, Cover-ups, and Winning at All Costs*. 1st ed. New York: Bantam Books.

Handyside, AH, JG Lesko, JJ Tarin, Robert Winston, and Mark Hughes. 1992. "Birth of a Normal Girl after in Vitro Fertilization and Preimplantation Diagnostic Testing for Cystic Fibrosis." *The New England Journal of Medicine* 327 (13): 905–09.

Harper, J C, L Wilton, J Traeger-Synodinos, V Goossens, C Moutou, S B SenGupta, T Pehlivan Budak, et al. 2012. "The ESHRE PGD

Consortium: 10 Years of Data Collection." *Human Reproduction Update* 18 (3) (June): 234–247. doi:10.1093/humupd/dmr052.

Harridge, Stephen D.R., and Cristiana P. Velloso. 2008. "Gene Doping." *Essays in Biochemistry* 44 (1) (December 1): 125. doi:10.1042/ BSE0440125.

Harris, J, and S Chan. 2008. "Enhancement Is Good for You!: Understanding the Ethics of Genetic Enhancement." *Gene Therapy* 15 (5) (January 24): 338–339. doi:10.1038/sj.gt.3303101.

Harris, John. (2005). No sex selection please, we're British. Journal of medical ethics, 31(5), 286-288.

———.. 2005. "Reproductive Liberty, Disease and Disability." *Reproductive Biomedicine Online* 10 Suppl 1 (March): 13–16.

———. 2007. *Enhancing Evolution the Ethical Case for Making Better People.* Princeton, NJ: Princeton University Press. http://public.eblib.com/ EBLPublic/PublicView.do?ptiID=457817.

———. 2011. "The Challenge of Nonconfrontational Ethics." *Cambridge Quarterly of Healthcare Ethics* 20 (02) (March 25): 204–215. doi:10.1017/ S096318011000085X.

Häyry, Matti. 2010. *Rationality and the Genetic Challenge: Making People Better?* Cambridge Law, Medicine, and Ethics. Cambridge, UK ; New York: Cambridge University Press.

Henderson, Gail E, Michele M Easter, Catherine Zimmer, Nancy M P King, Arlene M Davis, Barbra Bluestone Rothschild, Larry R Churchill, Benjamin S Wilfond, and Daniel K Nelson. 2006. "Therapeutic Misconception in Early Phase Gene Transfer Trials." *Social Science & Medicine (1982)* 62 (1) (January): 239–253. doi:10.1016/j. socscimed.2005.05.022.

HFEA. 2002. "Sex Selection: Options for Regulations." http://www.hfea. gov.uk/docs/Final_sex_selection_summary.pdf.

———. 2013. "List of HFEA Conditions Approved for PGD." http:// www.hfea.gov.uk/cps/hfea/gen/pgd-screening.htm.

HFEA Act. 2008 http://www.hfea.gov.uk/134.html (accessed March 18, 2014)

Hilgert, Nele, Richard J H Smith, and Guy Van Camp. 2009. "Forty-six Genes Causing Nonsyndromic Hearing Impairment: Which Ones

Should Be Analyzed in DNA Diagnostics?" *Mutation Research* 681 (2-3) (June): 189–196. doi:10.1016/j.mrrev.2008.08.002.

Hoberman, John. 2009. "Putting Doping into Context." In *Performance-enhancing Technologies in Sports: Ethical, Conceptual, and Scientific Issues*, edited by Thomas H. Murray, Karen J. Maschke, and Angela A. Wasunna. Baltimore: Johns Hopkins University Press.

Hollon, T. 2000. "Researchers and Regulators Reflect on First Gene Therapy Death." *Nature Medicine* 6 (1) (January): 6. doi:10.1038/71545.

Holm, Søren. 2007. "Doping Under Medical Control – Conceptually Possible but Impossible in the World of Professional Sports?" *Sport, Ethics and Philosophy* 1 (2) (August): 135–145. doi:10.1080/17511320701425116.

Horng, Sam, and Christine Grady. 2003. "Misunderstanding in Clinical Research: Distinguishing Therapeutic Misconception, Therapeutic Misestimation, and Therapeutic Optimism." *IRB* 25 (1) (February): 11–16.

Howe, P. David. 2004. *Sport, Professionalism, and Pain: Ethnographies of Injury and Risk*. London; New York: Routledge.

Huizenga, Rob. 1995. *"You're OK, It's Just a Bruise": a Doctor's Sideline Secrets About Pro Football's Most Outrageous Team*. New York: St. Martin's Griffin.

Hurley, J, S Birch, G Stoddart, and G Torrance. 1997. "Medical Necessity, Benefit and Resource Allocation in Health Care." *Journal of Health Services Research & Policy* 2 (4) (October): 223–230.

Johnson, Corey G. 2013. "Female Inmates Sterilized in California Prisons Without Approval". Center for Investigative Reporting. http://cironline.org/reports/female-inmates-sterilized-california-prisons-without-approval-4917.

Kakuk, Péter. 2008. "Gene Concepts and Genethics: Beyond Exceptionalism." *Science and Engineering Ethics* 14 (3) (September): 357–375. doi:10.1007/s11948-008-9056-7.

Karkazis, Katrina, Rebecca Jordan-Young, Georgiann Davis, and Silvia Camporesi. 2012. "Out of Bounds? A Critique of the New Policies on Hyperandrogenism in Elite Female Athletes." *The American Journal of Bioethics: AJOB* 12 (7): 3–16. doi:10.1080/15265161.2012.680533.

Kass, Leon. 2002. *Life, Liberty, and the Defense of Dignity: The Challenge for*

Bioethics. 1st ed. San Francisco: Encounter Books.

Kim, Hyun-Joong, Shin Yi Jang, Joong-Il Park, Jonghoe Byun, Dong-Ik Kim, Young-Soo Do, Jong-Mook Kim, et al. 2004. "Vascular Endothelial Growth Factor-induced Angiogenic Gene Therapy in Patients with Peripheral Artery Disease." *Experimental & Molecular Medicine* 36 (4) (August 31): 336–344.

Kimmelman, Jonathan. 2010. *Gene Transfer and the Ethics of First-in-human Research: Lost in Translation*. Cambridge, UK ; New York: Cambridge University Press.

Kimmelman, Jonathan, and Aaron Levenstadt. 2005. "Elements of Style: Consent Form Language and the Therapeutic Misconception in Phase 1 Gene Transfer Trials." *Human Gene Therapy* 16 (4) (April): 502–508. doi:10.1089/hum.2005.16.502.

King, Nancy M. P., and Richard Robeson. 2007. "Athlete or Guinea Pig? Sports and Enhancement Research." *Studies in Ethics, Law, and Technology* 1 (1) (January 21). doi:10.2202/1941-6008.1006. http://www.degruyter.com/view/j/selt.2007.1.1/selt.2007.1.1.1006/selt.2007.1.1.1006.xml.

———. 2013. "Athletes Are Guinea Pigs." *The American Journal of Bioethics* 13 (10) (October): 13–14. doi:10.1080/15265161.2013.828126.

Koessler, K. 2006. "Sport and the Psychology of Pain." In *Pain and Injury in Sport: Social and Ethical Analysis*, edited by Sigmund Loland, Berit Skirstad, and Ivan Waddington, 34–48. Ethics and Sport. London ; New York: Routledge.

Kotz, Deborah. 2012. "Boston Researchers Find New Evidence Linking Repeat Concussions to Permanent Brain Injury." *Boston.com*, December 2. http://www.boston.com/lifestyle/health/2012/12/03/boston-researchers-find-new-evidence-linking-repeat-concussions-permanent-brain-injury/qvJNGvLChiDRQOC0xkIKUJ/story.html.

Krumer, Alex, Tal Shavit, and Mosit Rosenboim. 2011. "Why Do Professional Athletes Have Different Time Preferences Than Non-athletes?" *Judgment and Decision Making* 6 (6): 542–551.

Kruse, P, J Ladefoged, U Nielsen, P E Paulev, and J P Sørensen. 1986. "Beta-Blockade Used in Precision Sports: Effect on Pistol Shooting Performance." *Journal of Applied Physiology* 61 (2) (August): 417–420.

LaFollette, Hugh. 2010. "Licensing Parents Revisited: Licensing Parents

Revisited." *Journal of Applied Philosophy* 27 (4): 327–343. doi:10.1111/j.1468-5930.2010.00497.x.

LA Times Associated Press. 2003. "Panel Backs Use of Growth Hormone in Short but Healthy Kids." *Los Angeles Times*. http://articles.latimes.com/2003/jun/11/nation/na-growth11.

Lehrman, S. 1999. "Virus Treatment Questioned after Gene Therapy Death." *Nature* 401 (6753) (October 7): 517–518. doi:10.1038/43977.

Leuenberger, Nicolas, Christian Reichel, and Françoise Lasne. 2012. "Detection of Erythropoiesis-stimulating Agents in Human Anti-doping Control: Past, Present and Future." *Bioanalysis* 4 (13) (July): 1565–1575. doi:10.4155/bio.12.153.

Lev, Ori, FG Miller, and E J Emanuel. 2010. "The Ethics of Research on Enhancement Interventions." *Kennedy Institute of Ethics Journal* 20 (2): 101–113. doi:10.1353/ken.0.0314.

Levi Setti, P E, E Albani, M Matteo, E Morenghi, E Zannoni, A M Baggiani, V Arfuso, and P Patrizio. 2013. "Five Years (2004-2009) of a Restrictive Law-regulating ART in Italy Significantly Reduced Delivery Rate: Analysis of 10,706 Cycles." *Human Reproduction (Oxford, England)* 28 (2) (February): 343–349. doi:10.1093/humrep/des404.

Levy, N. 2002. "Deafness, Culture, and Choice." *Journal of Medical Ethics* 28 (5): 284–285. doi:10.1136/jme.28.5.284.

Lewens, Tim. 2009. "Enhancement and Human Nature: The Case of Sandel." *Journal of Medical Ethics* 35 (6) (May 29): 354–356. doi:10.1136/jme.2008.028423.

Li, Zicong, Baoping Zhao, Yong Soo Kim, Ching Yuan Hu, and Jinzeng Yang. 2010. "Administration of a Mutated Myostatin Propeptide to Neonatal Mice Significantly Enhances Skeletal Muscle Growth." *Molecular Reproduction and Development* 77 (1) (January): 76–82. doi:10.1002/mrd.21111.

Lindemann, Hilde. 1997. *Stories and Their Limits: Narrative Approaches to Bioethics*. Reflective Bioethics. New York: Routledge.

Little, Maggie Olivia. 1998. "Cosmetic Surgery, Suspect Norms, and the Ethics of Complicity." In *Enhancing Human Traits: Ethical and Social Implications*, edited by Parens, Erik, 162–176. Georgetown University Press.

Loland, Sigmund. 2002. *Fair Play in Sport: a Moral Norm System*. Ethics and Sport. London ; New York: Routledge.

———. 2009. "Fairness in Sport: An Ideal and Its Consequences." In *Performance-enhancing Technologies in Sports: Ethical, Conceptual, and Scientific Issues*, edited by Thomas H. Murray, Karen J. Maschke, and Angela A. Wasunna, 175–204. Baltimore: Johns Hopkins University Press.

Loland, Sigmund, and Hans Hoppeler. 2012. "Justifying Anti-doping: The Fair Opportunity Principle and the Biology of Performance Enhancement." *European Journal of Sport Science* 12 (4) (July): 347–353. do i:10.1080/17461391.2011.566374.

Lombardo, Paul A. 2011. *A Century of Eugenics in America: From the Indiana Experiment to the Human Genome Era*. Bioethics and the Humanities. Bloomington, Ind: Indiana University Press.

Lotz, Mianna. 2006. "Feinberg, Mills, and the Child's Right to an Open Future." *Journal of Social Philosophy* 37 (4) (December): 537–551. doi:10.1111/j.1467-9833.2006.00356.x.

Lurie, Y. 2006. "The Ontology of Sport Injuries." In *Pain and Injury in Sport: Social and Ethical Analysis*, edited by Sigmund Loland, Berit Skirstad, and Ivan Waddington, 200–211. Ethics and Sport. London ; New York: Routledge.

Luzzatto, L. 1981. "[Thalassemia and malaria selection]." *Minerva medica* 72 (10) (March 17): 603–612.

MacArthur, Daniel. 2008. "The ACTN3 Sports Gene Test: What Can It Really Tell You?" *Wired*, November 30. http://www.wired.com/wiredscience/2008/11/the-actn3-sports-gene-test-what-can-it-really-tell-you/.

Macedo, Antero, Manuela Moriggi, Michele Vasso, Sara De Palma, Mauro Sturnega, Giorgio Friso, Cecilia Gelfi, Mauro Giacca, and Serena Zacchigna. 2012. "Enhanced Athletic Performance on Multisite AAV-IGF1 Gene Transfer Coincides with Massive Modification of the Muscle Proteome." *Human Gene Therapy* 23 (2) (February): 146–157. doi:10.1089/hum.2011.157.

MacIntyre, Alasdair C. 1984. *After Virtue: a Study in Moral Theory*. 2nd ed. Notre Dame, Ind: University of Notre Dame Press.

Mackenzie, Catriona, and Jackie Leach Scully. 2007. "Moral Imagination,

Disability and Embodiment." *Journal of Applied Philosophy* 24 (4) (November): 335–351. doi:10.1111/j.1468-5930.2007.00388.x.

MacMullan, Jackie. 2013. "Kobe Bryant Pushes Onward." *ESPN Boston*, February 7. http://espn.go.com/los-angeles/nba/story/_/id/8924518/kobe-bryant-tries-push-los-angeles-lakers-frustration.

Macur, Juliet. 2008. "Born to Run? Little Ones Get Test for Sports Gene." *The New York Times*, November 29. http://www.nytimes.com/2008/11/30/sports/30genetics.html?_r=0.

Maggiorelli, Simona. 2012. "Legge 40, Il Governo Monti Ricorre Contro La Sentenza Della Corte Europea Dei Diritti Dell'uomo." *Left*, November 28. http://www.left.it/2012/11/28/legge-40-il-governo-monti-ricorre-contro-la-sentenza-della-corte-di-strasburgo/7682/.

Mameli, M. 2007. "Reproductive Cloning, Genetic Engineering and the Autonomy of the Child: The Moral Agent and the Open Future." *Journal of Medical Ethics* 33 (2): 87–93. doi:10.1136/jme.2006.016634.

Manna, Claudio, and Luciano G Nardo. 2005. "Italian Law on Assisted Conception: Clinical and Research Implications." *Reproductive Biomedicine Online* 11 (5) (November): 532–534.

Mansour, Mai M. H., and Hassan M. E. Azzazy. 2009. "The Hunt for Gene Dopers." *Drug Testing and Analysis* 1 (7): 311–322. doi:10.1002/dta.52.

Maranto, Gina. 2013. "Meet the New Eugenics, Same as the Old Eugenics." *Biopolitical Times*. http://www.biopoliticaltimes.org/article.php?id=6725.

Mathias, Michael B. 2004. "The Competing Demands of Sport and Health: An Essay on the History of Ethics in Sports Medicine." *Clinics in Sports Medicine* 23 (2) (April): 195–214, vi. doi:10.1016/j.csm.2004.02.001.

McCabe, Linda L., and Edward R.B. McCabe. 2011. "Are We Entering a 'Perfect Storm' for a Resurgence of Eugenics? Science, Medicine and Their Social Context." In *A Century of Eugenics in America: From the Indiana Experiment to the Human Genome Era*, edited by Paul A. Lombardo, 193–218. Bioethics and the Humanities. Bloomington, Ind: Indiana University Press.

McCarthy, D. 2001. Why sex selection should be legal. Journal of Medical Ethics, 27(5), 302-307.

McFarlane, Craig, Gu Zi Hui, Wong Zhi Wei Amanda, Hiu Yeung Lau, Sudarsanareddy Lokireddy, Ge Xiaojia, Vincent Mouly, et al. 2011.

"Human Myostatin Negatively Regulates Human Myoblast Growth and Differentiation." *American Journal of Physiology. Cell Physiology* 301 (1) (July): C195–203. doi:10.1152/ajpcell.00012.2011.

McGrath, M. 2012. "Is Pain Medication in Sports a Form of Legal Doping?" *BBC News Science and Environment* (June 4). http://www.bbc.co.uk/news/science-environment-18282072.

McKanna, Trudy A., and Helga V. Toriello. 2010. "Gene Doping: The Hype and the Harm." *Pediatric Clinics of North America* 57 (3): 719–727. doi:10.1016/j.pcl.2010.02.006.

McLean, Sean. 2013. "Steroid Era Continues to Affect Major League Baseball." *UMass Boston*, August 26. http://www.umassmedia.com/sports/steroid-era-continues-to-affect-major-league-baseball/article_aa0ba342-0eb2-11e3-b91f-0019bb30f31a.html.

McNamee, M J. 2012. "The Spirit of Sport and the Medicalisation of Anti-Doping: Empirical and Normative Ethics." *Asian Bioethics Review* 4 (4): 347–392.

McNamee, M. J, and L. Tarasti. 2010. "Juridical and Ethical Peculiarities in Doping Policy." *Journal of Medical Ethics* 36 (3) (March 8): 165–169. doi:10.1136/jme.2009.030023.

McNamee, M. J. 2008. *Sports, Virtues and Vices: Morality Plays*. London ; New York: Routledge.

McNamee, M.J. 2006. "Suffering in and for Sport: Some Philosophical Remarks on a Painful Emotion." In *Pain and Injury in Sport: Social and Ethical Analysis*, edited by Sigmund Loland, Berit Skirstad, and Ivan Waddington, 229–45. Ethics and Sport. London ; New York: Routledge.

McNamee, Michael John, Arno Müller, Ivo van Hilvoorde, and Søren Holm. 2009. "Genetic Testing and Sports Medicine Ethics." *Sports Medicine* 39 (5): 339–344. doi:10.2165/00007256-200939050-00001.

Meghani, Zahra. 2011. "A Robust, Particularist Ethical Assessment of Medical Tourism." *Developing World Bioethics* 11 (1) (April): 16–29. doi:10.1111/j.1471-8847.2010.00282.x.

Mehlmann, Maxwell J. 2011. "Modern Eugenics and the Law." In *A Century of Eugenics in America: From the Indiana Experiment to the Human Genome Era*, edited by Paul A. Lombardo, 219–240. Bioethics and the Humanities. Bloomington, Ind: Indiana University Press.

Menuz, Vincent, Thierry Hurlimann, and Béatrice Godard. 2011. "Is Human Enhancement Also a Personal Matter?" *Science and Engineering Ethics* 19 (1): 161–177. doi:10.1007/s11948-011-9294-y.

Miah, Andy. 2006. "Rethinking Enhancement in Sport." *Annals of the New York Academy of Sciences* 1093 (December): 301–320. doi:10.1196/annals.1382.020.

Middleton, A, J Hewison, and R F Mueller. 1998. "Attitudes of Deaf Adults Toward Genetic Testing for Hereditary Deafness." *American Journal of Human Genetics* 63 (4): 1175–1180. doi:10.1086/302060.

Miller, Seumas, and Michael J. Selgelid. 2007. "Ethical and Philosophical Consideration of the Dual-use Dilemma in the Biological Sciences." *Science and Engineering Ethics* 13 (4): 523–580. doi:10.1007/s11948-007-9043-4.

Mills, Claudia. 2003. "The Child's Right to an Open Future?" *Journal of Social Philosophy* 34 (4) (December): 499–509. doi:10.1111/1467-9833.00197.

Mughal, N A, D A Russell, S Ponnambalam, and S Homer-Vanniasinkam. 2012. "Gene Therapy in the Treatment of Peripheral Arterial Disease." *The British Journal of Surgery* 99 (1) (January): 6–15. doi:10.1002/bjs.7743.

Mundy, Liza. 2002. "A World of Their Own." *The Washington Post*, March 31. http://wcfcourier.com/a-world-of-their-own/article_571dcc9e-860e-56df-80eb-03c2c2d474d6.html.

Muona, K, K Mäkinen, M Hedman, H Manninen, and S Ylä-Herttuala. 2012. "10-year Safety Follow-up in Patients with Local VEGF Gene Transfer to Ischemic Lower Limb." *Gene Therapy* 19 (4) (April): 392–395. doi:10.1038/gt.2011.109.

Murray, Thomas H. 2009a. "Ethics and Endurance-enhancing Technologies in Sport." In *Performance-enhancing Technologies in Sports: Ethical, Conceptual, and Scientific Issues*, edited by Thomas H. Murray, Karen J. Maschke, and Angela A. Wasunna, 155–. Baltimore: Johns Hopkins University Press.

Murray, Thomas H. 2009b. "In Search of an Ethics for Sport: Genetic Hierarchies, Handicappers General, and Embodied Excellence." In *Performance-enhancing Technologies in Sports: Ethical, Conceptual, and Scientific Issues*, edited by Thomas H. Murray, Karen J. Maschke, and Angela A. Wasunna. Baltimore: Johns Hopkins University Press.

Naish, John. 2012. "Genetically Modified Athletes: Forget Drugs. There Are

Even Suggestions Some Chinese Athletes' Genes Are Altered to Make Them Stronger." *Daily Mail*, August 1. http://www.dailymail.co.uk/ news/article-2181873/Genetically-modified-athletes-Forget-drugs-There-suggestions-Chinese-athletes-genes-altered-make-stronger.html.

National Research Council. 2013. *An Ecosystem Services Approach to Assessing the Impacts of the Deepwater Horizon Oil Spill in the Gulf of Mexico.* Washington, D.C: The National Academies Press.

National Task Force on CME. 2013. "On-label and Off-label Usage of Prescription Medicines and Devices, and the Relationship to Continuing Medical Education." http://www.ama-assn.org/resources/doc/cme/ fact-sheet-4.pdf.

Nixon, H. L. 1992. "A Social Network Analysys of Influences On Athletes To Play With Pain and Injuries." *Journal of Sport & Social Issues* 16 (2) (September 1): 127–135. doi:10.1177/019372359201600208.

———. 1993. "Accepting the Risks of Pain and Injury in Sports; Mediated Cultural Influences on Playing Hurt." *Sociology of Sport Journal* 13: 127–135.

Ohlheiser, Abby. 2013. "California Prisons Were Illegally Sterilizing Female Inmates." *The Atlantic Wire*, July 7. http://www.theatlanticwire.com/ national/2013/07/california-prisons-were-illegally-sterilizing-female-inmates/66905/.

Oliver, Michael. 1996. *Understanding Disability: From Theory to Practice.* 2nd ed. Basingstoke, Hampshire [England] ; New York: Palgrave Macmillan.

Østergård, T, J Ek, Y Hamid, B Saltin, O B Pedersen, T Hansen, and O Schmitz. 2005. "Influence of the PPAR-gamma2 Pro12Ala and ACE I/D Polymorphisms on Insulin Sensitivity and Training Effects in Healthy Offspring of Type 2 Diabetic Subjects." *Hormone and Metabolic Research = Hormon- Und Stoffwechselforschung = Hormones et Métabolisme* 37 (2) (February): 99–105. doi:10.1055/s-2005-861174.

Ostrander, Elaine A, Heather J Huson, and Gary K Ostrander. 2009. "Genetics of Athletic Performance." *Annual Review of Genomics and Human Genetics* 10: 407–429. doi:10.1146/annurev-genom-082908-150058.

Parens, Erik. 1998. "Special Supplement: Is Better Always Good? The Enhancement Project." *The Hastings Center Report* 28 (1) (January): S1.

doi:10.2307/3527981.

———. 2005. "Authenticity and Ambivalence: Toward Understanding the Enhancement Debate." *The Hastings Center Report* 35 (3) (June): 34–41.

Parens, Erik, and Adrienne Asch. 2000. *Prenatal Testing and Disability Rights.* Hastings Center Studies in Ethics. Washington, D.C: Georgetown University Press.

Parfit, Derek. 1984. *Reasons and Persons.* Oxford [Oxfordshire]: Clarendon Press.

"Petition Against Clause 14(4)(9) of HFE Bill and Government Response." 2008. http://www.grumpyoldeafies.com/2008/05/petition_against_1449_human_fe.html.

Porter, Dorothy Elizabeth. 2011. *Health Citizenship: Essays in Social Medicine and Biomedical Politics.* Perspectives in Medical Humanities 5. San Francisco, CA: University of California Medical Humanities Press.

Practice Committee of the ASRM. 2006. "Preimplantation Genetic Diagnosis." *Fertility and Sterility* 86 (5 Suppl 1): S257–258. doi:10.1016/j.fertnstert.2006.08.028.

President's Council on Bioethics (U.S.). 2003. *Beyond Therapy: Biotechnology and the Pursuit of Happiness.* 1st ed. New York: ReganBooks.

Rawls, John. 1971. *A Theory of Justice.* Original ed. Cambridge, Mass: Belknap Press.

Resnik, David B. 2000. "The Moral Significance of the Therapy-enhancement Distinction in Human Genetics." *Cambridge Quarterly of Healthcare Ethics: CQ: The International Journal of Healthcare Ethics Committees* 9 (3): 365–377.

Reynolds, Emma. 2012. "London 2012 Unveils Anti-doping Laboratory." http://www.kcl.ac.uk/newsevents/news/newsrecords/2012/01Jan/London-2012-unveil-Anti-Doping-Laboratory.aspx.

Reynolds, Gretchen. 2007. "Outlaw DNA." *The New York Times.* http://www.nytimes.com/2007/06/03/sports/playmagazine/0603play-hot.html?pagewanted=all&_r=0.

Roberts, Dorothy. 2000. "Forum: Black Women and the Pill." *Family Planning Perspectives* 32 (2). http://www.guttmacher.org/pubs/journals/3209200.html.

Robertson, John A. 2003. "Procreative Liberty in the Era of Genomics."

American Journal of Law & Medicine 29: 439–87.

Roth, Stephen M. 2012. "Critical Overview of Applications of Genetic Testing in Sport Talent Identification." *Recent Patents on DNA & Gene Sequences* 6 (3) (December): 247–255.

Rothman, Sheila M., and David J. Rothman. 2003. *The Pursuit of Perfection: The Promise and Perils of Medical Enhancement.* 1st ed. New York: Pantheon Books.

Rozmus, Alexander. 2013. "Canada: Modernizing Liability For Offshore Oil & Gas Explorations And Operations." *Mondaq*, August 18. http://www.mondaq.com/canada/x/258476/Oil+Gas+Electricity/Modernizing+Liability+For+Offshore+Oil+amp+Gas+Explorations+And+Operations.

Rupert, J L. 2009. "Transcriptional Profiling: a Potential Anti-doping Strategy." *Scandinavian Journal of Medicine & Science in Sports* 19 (6) (December): 753–763. doi:10.1111/j.1600-0838.2009.00970.x.

Sadler, John Z. 2010. "Dignity, *Arête* , and Hubris in the Transhumanist Debate." *The American Journal of Bioethics* 10 (7) (June 30): 67–68. doi:10.1080/15265161003728845.

Sandel, Michael. 2004. "The Case Against Perfection." *The Athlantic.* http://www.theatlantic.com/magazine/archive/2004/04/the-case-against-perfection/302927/.

Sanghavi, D.M. 2006. "Wanting Babies Like Themselves, Some Parents Choose Genetic Defects." *New York Times* (December 5). http://www.nytimes.com/2006/12/05/health/05essa.html?_r=0.

Savulescu, J, Bennett Foddy, and M. Clayton. 2004. "Why We Should Allow Performance Enhancing Drugs in Sport." *British Journal of Sports Medicine* 38 (6) (December 1): 666–670. doi:10.1136/bjsm.2003.005249.

Savulescu, Julian. 2006. "Justice, Fairness, and Enhancement." *Annals of the New York Academy of Sciences* 1093 (1) (December 1): 321–338. doi:10.1196/annals.1382.021.

———. 2013. "Time to Rethink Case for Legalised Doping." *The New Zealand Herald*, July 20. http://www.nzherald.co.nz/sport/news/article.cfm?c_id=4&objectid=10900371.

———.. 2009. "Genetic Interventions and the Ethics of Enhancement of Human Beings." In *Readings in the Philosophy of Technology*, 2nd Edition, 417–430. Rowman & Littlefield Publishers.

Schapiro, Tamar. 1999. "What Is a Child?" *Ethics* 109 (4) (July): 715–738. doi:10.1086/233943.

Schwarz, Alan. 2009. "Dementia Risk Seen in Players in N.F.L. Study." *The New York Times*, September 29. http://www.nytimes.com/2009/09/30/sports/football/30dementia.html?pagewanted=all&_r=1&.

Scripko, P. D. 2010. "Enhancement's Place in Medicine." *Journal of Medical Ethics* 36 (5) (May 3): 293–296. doi:10.1136/jme.2009.032383.

Scully, Jackie Leach. 2008. "Disability and Genetics in the Era of Genomic Medicine." *Nature Reviews Genetics* 9 (10) (October): 797–802. doi:10.1038/nrg2453.

Segerson, Kathleen, and Tom Tietenberg. 1992. "The Structure of Penalties in Environmental Enforcement: An Economic Analysis." *Journal of Environmental Economics and Management* 23: 179–200.

Selgelid, Michael J. 2009. "A Moderate Pluralist Approach to Public Health Policy and Ethics." *Public Health Ethics* 2 (2) (July 3): 195–205. doi:10.1093/phe/php018.

———. 2012. "A Moderate Approach To Enhancement." *Philosophy Now* (91) (August). http://philosophynow.org/issues/91/A_Moderate_Approach_To_Enhancement.

———. 2013. "Moderate Eugenics and Human Enhancement." *Medicine, Health Care and Philosophy* (June 1). doi:10.1007/s11019-013-9485-1. http://link.springer.com/10.1007/s11019-013-9485-1.

SenGupta, Sioban B, and Joy D A Delhanty. 2012. "Preimplantation Genetic Diagnosis: Recent Triumphs and Remaining Challenges." *Expert Review of Molecular Diagnostics* 12 (6) (July): 585–592. doi:10.1586/erm.12.61.

Shakespeare, Tom. 2013. *Disability Rights and Wrongs Revisited.*

Silver, Lee M. 1997. *Remaking Eden: Cloning and Beyond in a Brave New World.* 1st ed. New York: Avon Books.

Silver, M D. 2001. "Use of Ergogenic Aids by Athletes." *The Journal of the American Academy of Orthopaedic Surgeons* 9 (1) (February): 61–70.

Slote, Michael A. 1989. *Goods and Virtues.* Oxford: Clarendon Press.

Soini, S. 2007. "Preimplantation Genetic Diagnosis (PGD) in Europe: Diversity of Legislation a Challenge to the Community and Its Citizens." *Medicine and Law* 26 (2) (June): 309–323.

Solomon, Andrew. 2012. *Far from the Tree: Parents, Children and the Search for*

Identity. New York: Scribner.

Sparrow, Rob. 2011. "A Not-So-New Eugenics: Harris and Savulescu on HumanEnhancement," *Hastings Center Report* 41 (1): 32–42.

Spriggs, M. 2002. "Lesbian Couple Create a Child Who Is Deaf Like Them." *Journal of Medical Ethics* 28 (5) (October): 283.

Springer, M L, A S Chen, P E Kraft, M Bednarski, and H M Blau. 1998. "VEGF Gene Delivery to Muscle: Potential Role for Vasculogenesis in Adults." *Molecular Cell* 2 (5) (November): 549–558.

Stein, Rob. 2011. "Genetic Testing for Sports Generates Controversy, Genetic Testing for Sports Genes Courts Controversy." *The Washington Post*, May 18. http://www.washingtonpost.com/national/genetic-testing-for-sports-genes-courts-controversy/2011/05/09/AFkTuV6G_story.html.

Stern, S J, K S Arnos, L Murrelle, K Oelrich Welch, W E Nance, and A Pandya. 2002. "Attitudes of Deaf and Hard of Hearing Subjects Towards Genetic Testing and Prenatal Diagnosis of Hearing Loss." *Journal of Medical Genetics* 39 (6) (June): 449–453.

Straubel, Michael S. 2002. "Doping Due Process: A Critique of the Doping Control Process in International Sport." *Dickinson Law Review* 106: 523–31.

Sullivan, Nora. 2013. "California Uses Tax Funds to Illegally Sterilize 148 Inmates." *Life News*, July 7. http://www.lifenews.com/2013/07/10/california-uses-tax-funds-to-illegally-sterilize-148-inmates/.

Sullivan, Richard, Jeffrey Peppercorn, Karol Sikora, John Zalcberg, Neal J Meropol, Eitan Amir, David Khayat, et al. 2011. "Delivering Affordable Cancer Care in High-income Countries." *The Lancet Oncology* 12 (10) (September): 933–980. doi:10.1016/S1470-2045(11)70141-3.

Suter, Sonia. 2007. "A Brave New World of Designer Babies." *Berkeley Technology Law Journal* 22 (897): 897–969.

Tannsjo, T. 2005. "Hypoxic Air Machines. Commentary." *Journal of Medical Ethics* 31 (2) (February 1): 113–113. doi:10.1136/jme.2003.005355.

———. 2010. "Medical Enhancement and the Ethos of Elite Sport." In *Human Enhancement*, edited by Julian Savulescu and Nick Bostrom, 315–26. Oxford: Oxford University Press.

Tauer, Carol A. 1994. "The NIH Trials of Growth Hormone for Short

Stature." *IRB* 16 (3): 1–9.

Telegraph Staff. 2010. "London 2012 Olympics: Wada Hails Drug Breakthrough to Combat Cheats." *Telegraph*, September 4. http://www. telegraph.co.uk/sport/olympics/7981501/London-2012-Olympics-Wada-hails-drug-breakthrough-to-combat-cheats.html.

The Guardian Associated Press. 2013. "Lance Armstrong Settles with Sunday Times." *The Guardian*, August 25. http://www.theguardian.com/sport/2013/aug/25/lance-armstrong-settles-sunday-times.

Tracey, Irene, and M. Catherine Bushnell. 2009. "How Neuroimaging Studies Have Challenged Us to Rethink: Is Chronic Pain a Disease?" *The Journal of Pain* 10 (11) (November): 1113–1120. doi:10.1016/j.jpain.2009.09.001.

Tuffs, A. 2011. "Germany Allows Restricted Access to Preimplantation Genetic Testing." *BMJ* 343 (jul12 1) (July 12): d4425–d4425. doi:10.1136/bmj.d4425.

Turone, F. 2012. "European Court Overturns Preimplantation Testing Ban." *BMJ* 345 (sep05 2) (September 5): e5996–e5996. doi:10.1136/bmj.e5996.

United Nations. 1992. "Rio Declaration on Environment and Development." http://www.jus.uio.no/lm/environmental.development.rio. declaration.1992/portrait.a4.pdf.

WADA Code. 2009. "World Anti-Doping Code." http://www.wada-ama. org/Documents/World_Anti-Doping_Program/WADP-The-Code/WADA_Anti-Doping_CODE_2009_EN.pdf.

———. 2012. "WADA Code." http://www.wada-ama.org/Documents/World_Anti-Doping_Program/WADP-IS-Testing/2012/WADA_IST_2012_EN.pdf.

WADA Official Publication Play True. 2007. "Gene Doping. An Overview and Update." *Play True* (2): 12–14.

WADA Official Publication Play True. 2008. "Levelling the Playing Field." (3): 19–24.

Waldron, Jennifer J., and Vikki Krane. 2005. "Whatever It Takes: Health Compromising Behaviors in Female Athletes." *Quest* 57 (3): 315–329. doi:10.1080/00336297.2005.10491860.

Wales Online. 2008. "Fears over Fertilisation and Embryology Bill Clause." *Wales Online*, April 7. http://www.walesonline.co.uk/news/health/fears-over-fertilisation-embryology-bill-2181367.

Wall, John. 2010. *Ethics in Light of Childhood*. Washington, D.C: Georgetown University Press.

Wearden, Graeme. 2010. "BP Oil Spill Costs to Hit $40bn." *The Guardian*, November 2. http://www.theguardian.com/business/2010/nov/02/bp-oil-spill-costs-40-billion-dollars.

Weinberg, Rick. 2004. "51: Kerri Strug Fights Off Pain, Helps U.S. Win Gold." *ESPN*. http://espn.go.com/espn/espn25/story?page=moments/51.

Wells, D J. 2008. "Gene Doping: The Hype and the Reality." *British Journal of Pharmacology* 154 (3) (June): 623–631. doi:10.1038/bjp.2008.144.

White, Hilary. 2012. "Italy Must Allow Embryo Genetic Screening Because of Unrestricted Abortion Law: Euro Court Ruling." *Lifesite Nes*, August 29. http://www.lifesitenews.com/news/italy-must-allow-embryo-genetic-screening-because-of-unrestricted-abortion/.

Wilens, Timothy E., Lenard A. Adler, Jill Adams, Stephanie Sgambati, John Rotrosen, Robert Sawtelle, Linsey Utzinger, and Steven Fusillo. 2008. "Misuse and Diversion of Stimulants Prescribed for ADHD: A Systematic Review of the Literature." *Journal of the American Academy of Child & Adolescent Psychiatry* 47 (1) (January): 21–31. doi:10.1097/chi.0b013e31815a56f1.

Wilkinson, S., & Garrard, E. 2013. Eugenics and the ethics of selective reproduction.http://eprints.lancs.ac.uk/65644/1/Eugenics_and_the_ethics_of_selective_reproduction_Low_Res_1.pdf (accessed March 18, 2014)

Wilson, James M. 2005. "Gendicine: The First Commercial Gene Therapy Product; Chinese Translation of Editorial." *Human Gene Therapy* 16 (9) (September): 1014–1015. doi:10.1089/hum.2005.16.1014.

Wilson, Michael P., and Megan R. Schwarzman. 2009. "Toward a New U.S. Chemicals Policy: Rebuilding the Foundation to Advance New Science, Green Chemistry and Environmental Health." *Environmental Health Perspectives*. doi:10.1289/ehp.0800404. http://ehp.niehs.nih.gov/docs/2009/0800404/abstract.html.

Winfrey, Oprah. 2013. "Lance Armstrong Talks to Oprah". Oprah Winfrey Network. http://www.oprah.com/own_tv/onc/lance-armstrong-one.html.

Wolff, Jonathan. 2011. *Ethics and Public Policy: a Philosophical Inquiry*. Milton Park, Abingdon, Oxon ; New York: Routledge.

Wolpe, Paul Root. 2002. "Treatment, Enhancement, and the Ethics of Neurotherapeutics." *Brain and Cognition* 50 (3): 387–395.

World Health Organization. 2001. "International Classification of Functioning, Disability and Health, 2001 Revision". WHO. http://www.who.int/classifications/icf/en/.

Yang, Nan, Daniel G MacArthur, Jason P Gulbin, Allan G Hahn, Alan H Beggs, Simon Easteal, and Kathryn North. 2003. "ACTN3 Genotype Is Associated with Human Elite Athletic Performance." *American Journal of Human Genetics* 73 (3) (September): 627–631. doi:10.1086/377590.

Zanini, Giulia. 2011. "Abandoned by the State, Betrayed by the Church: Italian Experiences of Cross-border Reproductive Care." *Reproductive BioMedicine Online* 23 (5) (November): 565–572. doi:10.1016/j.rbmo.2011.08.007.

Index